Mediterranean Diet:

A Complete guide with recipes and meal plan for weight loss

I0421356

Table of Contents

Mediterranean Diet Cookbook   (Book n.2)

Nessuna voce di sommario trovata.

Mediterranean Diet:

A Complete Guide and Recipe Inspirations

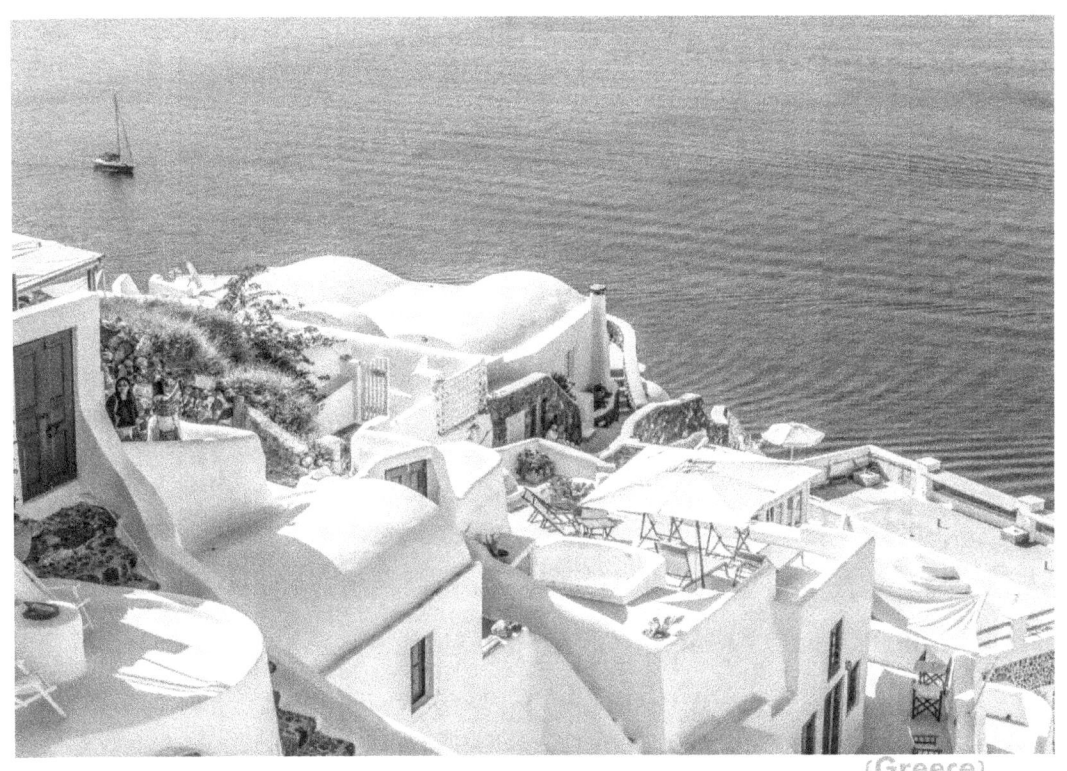

(Greece)

Introduction & Disclaimer

Congratulations and thank you for downloading *Mediterranean Diet*: A Complete Guide and Recipe Inspirations.

If you've been looking for the perfect diet to help improve your overall health and for you to lose weight as well, then the Mediterranean diet could be the answer! The U.S. News and World Report awarded this diet as the number one diet to try in 2019. This is because this diet focuses on fruits and vegetables, paired with lean meats and seafood to keep weight off and improve overall cardiovascular health. Along with decreases in blood sugar, cholesterol levels, and risk of cancer, this diet has become very popular mainly because it is very easy to do! You do not need to count carbs or keep track of your calories. Although you should still portion out your meals and try to maintain calorie deficit if you aim to lose weight, this diet is about changing what you eat instead of counting calories. It is a healthy and balanced lifestyle change that you can easily incorporate, as long as you remember what you can and cannot eat. For example, fish and seafood are encouraged at least a couple of times a week. Red meat, on the other hand, should be eaten occasionally and you should choose leaner cuts. Whole grains, fresh fruits and vegetables are also encouraged, along with making the switch to cooking with only olive oil.

Reviewing the scientific studies on the Mediterranean diet, it's easy to see why this diet has become so popular. The benefits regarding cardiovascular health alone are astounding, such as lowering cholesterol, improving heart strength, and lowering blood pressure. It has also been verified to stabilize blood sugar and prevent Type 2 diabetes for at-risk patients.

Couple this with other health benefits like fighting depression, improving sight, and improving mental alertness, this diet provides multiple health benefits that can reduce inflammation and improve longevity.

What appeals to many people is how easy this diet is! You don't have to count calories or macros, or portion out your meals. You should certainly be aware of portion sizes and what your caloric intake is, but the important thing is to adjust your diet so that you are eating healthier items and less red meat. From there, it's about living an active lifestyle which will help you lose excess weight.

In this book, we will explain the Mediterranean diet to you, give you insight to the science behind it and the health benefits you could gain. We will give you a typical shopping list of what to include and exclude when you are grocery shopping so you can stock up on healthy ingredients to prepare your meals. Along with a 14-day meal plan and snack ideas, this book will help you begin your Mediterranean diet and enjoy an array of delicious and healthy meals for breakfast, lunch, and dinner.

Before we begin, it is important that we state that this diet, and any other lifestyle changes should not be made without speaking to your personal doctor. Based on your individual medical history and medical needs, your doctor should approve any changes you make in your lifestyle and ensure they will not harm your condition or interfere with required medication. Your health is most important and it is required that you speak to your doctor regarding your individual health needs. If you have started the Mediterranean diet and then feel unwell, you should stop immediately and consult your physician on how to proceed.

There are plenty of books on this subject on the market, so thanks again for choosing this one!

Chapter 1: What is the Mediterranean Diet

The Mediterranean diet has become very popular in recent years with numerous studies to prove its health benefits. The diet is based on the traditional foods that people used to eat, and the lifestyle that they lived in countries of the Mediterranean throughout history. On a global scale, the residents of these areas were exceptionally healthier compared to Americans who may have multiple illnesses or shorter life spans. American scientist Ancel Keys noticed that the citizens living in poorer regions of Italy were overall healthier than the wealthiest New Yorkers. It was very common for farmers in the region of Greece to be nearly 100 years old! In the 1950s, Keys began a study between these populations and their diet choices. He established the connection between their lifestyle and their overall health by realizing the people of these regions were getting their fat intake from healthy fats like olive oil, nuts, and fresh fish. He also noted that this low saturated fat consumption resulted in fewer instances of heart disease and an overall longer life span. Although this research was conducted in the 1950s, the diet itself did not become popular in the United States until the late 1990s when it gained social following. It began to appeal to many because of how easy it was and how it did not require counting or keeping track of calories or macros.

By studying the diet and lifestyle of the people of those regions, the Mediterranean diet proved a healthier way of life that can produce weight loss results and other health benefits. What are some of these health benefits? The Mediterranean has proven to give followers a reduced risk of Type 2 diabetes and cardiovascular disease. It can even decrease the risk of having a heart attack, stroke, or suffering from premature death. That's right, you could even live longer by following this lifestyle!

Now, there are different ways of following the Mediterranean diet as there are many countries located around the Mediterranean Sea with many different foods. But by following one of their dietary patterns along with an active lifestyle, you can greatly improve your overall health and strengthen your heart as well. The general plan is more of a guideline where you can adjust it to your individual preferences and tastes.

What are the basic tenets of the Mediterranean diet to follow?

- **A diet full of:** vegetables (carrots, onions, spinach, garlic, broccoli, etc.) legumes (lentils, beans), whole grain breads & pasta, herbs, fish (salmon, sardines, trout, tilapia, mackerel, etc.), shrimp & seafood, extra virgin olive oil, nuts (almonds, cashews, walnuts, etc.), seeds (sunflower seeds, pumpkin seeds, etc.) , fruits (apples, oranges, grapes, bananas, berries, etc.), olives

- **Eat only in moderation:** cheese, eggs, poultry, yogurt

- **Eat rarely:** red meat

- **Avoid:** sugars (candy, sugary snacks), processed foods, refined grains (white bread or refined pasta), processed meat (packaged meat such as sausages, bacon, or hot dogs), refined oils (canola oil, soybean oil, and others), sweetened beverages (soda, sugary fruit juices)

Be sure to read the nutritional labels of new foods to ensure that they are not full of refined grains or are high in sugar. One of the important parts of the diet is using extra virgin olive oil for all cooking needs. You do not want to substitute this with a different, unhealthy type of cooking oil. Extra virgin olive oil is the unprocessed version of olive oil and contains high quality of compounds called phenols. These are known for their antioxidant qualities and lowering inflammation in the body. Olive oil also contains oleic acid which is heart-healthy compared to other oils or fats like butter or margarine. Most health practitioners recommend 3 to 4 tablespoons of olive oil a day. Always remember: you should use olive oil for all your cooking needs!

This diet is high in healthy plant foods and low in animal food like poultry and red meat. Instead, having seafood or fish at least twice a week is recommended. It's a great source of protein and packed with omega 3 fatty acids that are beneficial for your nerve cells and sight. Some critics say that the Mediterranean diet is too rich in fats and will only make you gain weight, but scientific studies show the opposite. It of course depends if you are eating calorie-deficit meals and if you are exercising.

Another aspect of the Mediterranean lifestyle is an active lifestyle. People sometimes focus so much on the dietary aspect that they don't realize how important exercise also is. A study found that engaging in just 30 minutes of moderate exercise multiple times a week can reduce the risk of early death by more than 25%! Simply being on the diet and hoping the weight will fall off and while you gain the health benefits is not enough. You have to mold your lifestyle to be successful, just as the people you are trying to emulate. The people of the Mediterranean led an active lifestyle at the time and many people often performed jobs requiring physical labor. Other than that, based on the coastal region, activities like swimming, sailing, rowing, and long walks were very common and reflected the daily exercise they would engage in. In the modern times, that means incorporating at least 20 to 30 minutes of moderate exercise a few times a week, whether that's jogging, walking, or low cardio.

How to Begin a Mediterranean Diet Lifestyle

If you're interested in following the Mediterranean diet lifestyle, we have some tips to help you get started!

Use healthy oils. One of the essential aspects of the Mediterranean lifestyle is using extra virgin olive oil. That means you need to replace any butter or unhealthy vegetable oils with extra virgin olive oil. You would want to use extra virgin olive oil in all your cooking, baking, frying, and even salad dressing. Even if it's just sautéing veggies, be sure you're using olive oil instead of butter.

Use more spices. If you're not one to use a lot of herbs and spices in your cooking, this is a great time to experiment and expand your palette. You want to try and reduce your salt intake and season your food with these dried herbs and spices to add flavor to your food. There's more out there than just salt and pepper! Try and experiment with new flavors and see how it can elevate your dish.

Allow natural sugars to be your dessert. We've gotten used to bake goods and sugary cakes as dessert options, but in many countries, they finish off the meal with fresh fruit or nuts. Instead of thinking of dessert as a forbidden option and tempting yourself even more, finish off your meals with some delicious and sweet friend, like orange slices, fresh berries, or melon. You have to change the notion that dessert has to be something unhealthy. Learn to satisfy your sweet tooth with healthy and natural options.

Re-think your meats. Instead of focusing on meals where steak or chicken is the star, try and have red meat and poultry less frequently throughout the month. Focus on having fish and seafood two or three times a week! There are many delicious options and ways that you can make fish and seafood into your meals, whether it's a stir fry, salad, tacos, or grilled. The health benefits that fish provides are also great to experience. It's filling and healthy without unnecessary fats.

Drink with your meals. If you are an avid wine drinker, then the Mediterranean diet is the one for you! Drinking wine with a meal is very common in countries around the Mediterranean Sea. This does not mean you're guzzling a few glasses during the day, but if you are going to have a glass, have it with your meal so you can gain the potential health benefits. This of course is not necessary if you are to avoid alcohol due to health reasons or are not a drinker. You can still follow the Mediterranean diet and gain the benefits.

Focus on what you can eat, not what you must avoid. Too many diets fail because people become trapped in what they cannot eat that it becomes so tempting to them! Though the Mediterranean diet has restrictions like we mentioned above, there are still so many options of what you can eat. Fruits, vegetables, beans, lentils, and seafood are all options that you can incorporate into your diet. Give yourself the chance to try these new foods and experiment with new recipes. When you start to explore and fall in love with these meals, you won't miss what you can't have.

Get active. If you still do not incorporate exercise into your lifestyle, it's important you do so now! People think of exercise as a chore and having to go the gym and take time out of their busy day. But truly becoming active does not necessarily mean you have to leave the comfort of your home. Whether it's following along to a video routine, gardening outside, going for a swim, or a bike ride around the neighborhood, there are so many ways to lead an active lifestyle.

Chapter 2: The Science Behind the Diet

Though the Mediterranean diet came from the lifestyle of the people of living in that indigenous area, the diet has only gained popularity in the recent decades in the West as a way to improve health and prevent disease. Since then, many scientific studies have been conducted with controlled variables to study the effects of this diet and the health benefits it can produce.

Here's a look at what some of the respected and peer-reviewed researches on the Mediterranean diet have found:

The PREDIMED Study: This study was conducted in 2013 and was made famous due to the results showing significant reductions in heart disease. It followed a large study of 7,447 individuals. They were randomized to one of three diet types: a low-fat control group, a Mediterranean diet with additional raw nut intake, and a Mediterranean diet with additional extra virgin olive oil. The study went on for almost 5 years and many papers have been written about the completed effects and reduction of risk factors. Here are some of the results that were found:

- The Mediterranean + Olive Oil group had a 30% decreased risk of suffering from a heart attack or stroke, while the Mediterranean + Nuts group had a 28% decrease. These results were more significant in male subjects, not female. People who had obesity, high blood pressure, and lipid problems tended to respond better to the Mediterranean diet.

- Individuals in both the Mediterranean diet groups had a decrease in oxidized LDL cholesterol while the low-fat control group did not have a statistically significant decrease.

- The Mediterranean diet groups were less likely to become diabetic in comparison to the control group that followed a low-fat diet. In the Mediterranean diet groups, 10% and 11% of individuals became diabetic, while nearly 18% of individuals in the low-fat control group had diabetes at the end of 4 years.

- After a 3-month study, the Mediterranean diet improved certain cardiovascular risk factors like high blood sugar levels, high HDL cholesterol ratio, high blood pressure, and C-Reactive Protein levels. The low-fat group again had no significant change.

- After 5 years, more than 300 people had died related to cardiovascular or cancer-related deaths. The group that consumed more nuts had anywhere from 16-65% lower risk of death during the study period.

Lyon Diet Heart Study: This 1999 study enrolled 605 middle-aged men and women who had previously suffered from a heart attack. They were split into two groups made to follow either a Mediterranean diet supplemented with Omega 3 fats or a more "conservative" Western style diet. After 4 years of study, it was found that the group that followed the Mediterranean lifestyle were more than 70% less likely to have died from heart disease or suffered from another heart attack.

- 4 people in the low-fat group had a stroke. 0 people did in the Mediterranean group.

The Journal of the American Medical Association: This 2004 study tested 180 patients with metabolic syndrome who were either following a more conservative diet or a Mediterranean diet. After 2.5 years of study, about 80% of the patients still had metabolic syndrome in the control group compared to less than 45% of patients in the Mediterranean diet group.

- The Mediterranean diet group also decreased their weight by nearly 10 pounds compared to only an average of 3 pounds weight loss in the control group.
- The Mediterranean diet group had significantly less inflammatory markers.
- The Mediterranean group followers had less insulin resistance than the control group followers.

The New England Journal of Medicine: 322 obese men and women were studied in 2008 to compare the Mediterranean diet to a low-fat and low carb diet. When total weight loss was assessed, the low-fat group lost only an average of 6 pounds while the Mediterranean diet group lost almost 10 pounds on average!

- The diet also improved blood sugar levels and insulin levels in the group who followed the Mediterranean diet.
- Losing weight on the Mediterranean diet also improves other diabetes risk signs like insulin resistance.
- After 4 years, less than half the Mediterranean diet group needed diabetes medication. The low-fat group had more than 70% of participants needing medication despite having followed their diet.
- A Mediterranean diet could delay the need for at risk diabetes patients to begin medication and prevent at risk patients from developing the disease. This is great news for people who have a family history of diabetes!

Even though the Mediterranean diet isn't necessarily prescribed for weight loss, it has been found that most participants tend to lose more weight compared to low carb or low-fat diets. This, coupled with reducing the cardiovascular disease risks, the Mediterranean diet could delay the onset of Type 2 diabetes, as excess weight is one of the symptoms of diabetes. The many research studies show that the Mediterranean diet is a more successful lifestyle change in controlling blood sugar levels than following a low-fat diet.

Chapter 3: The Incredible Health Benefits

A number of reasons explain why the Mediterranean Diet has been ranked #1 on U.S. News' Health ranking for 2018. It is relatively easy to follow, nutritious, essential in producing weight loss results, and gaining other overall health benefits. Don't take it from us - take it from the scientific experts! Numerous studies have found that consistently following a Mediterranean style diet can improve your health in many ways.

Here are some of the potential benefits you can gain!

Lowers risk of cardiovascular disease. The Mediterranean diet has been recognized to be the most helpful in reducing high triglyceride levels. These are the fatty molecules that travel throughout the bloodstream and build up plaque in our arteries. A higher triglyceride count can lead to higher cholesterol and an increased risk of stroke or heart attack. Even though the Mediterranean diet consists of fatty items like olive oil and salmon, these are good fats that are loaded with beneficial monounsaturated and polyunsaturated fats. A study tracked 28 men who ate Mediterranean diet meals for a week, followed by junk food meals for a week. They found that after the men had the Mediterranean meal, their arteries opened and they maintained a healthy blood flow. This was compared to after the junk food meal when their arteries failed to dilate and their blood flow function did not improve. The Mediterranean diet proves more effective at reducing high triglyceride counts, while still maintaining the presence of "good" cholesterol, or HDL cholesterol in the blood.

Improves heart health. A study shows that a Mediterranean diet rich in ALA (alpha linolenic acid) found in olive oil can decrease the risk of cardiac death in a person by nearly 30%[1]! Further research shows that when comparing the blood pressure between people who consumed sunflower oil versus those consuming extra virgin oil, the olive oil consumers were able to decrease their blood pressure by more significant amounts[2]. It might seem counterintuitive that olive oil can actually lower blood pressure, but using extra virgin olive oil keeps the oil unrefined which means the plant additions are intact and can improve cellular function. Couple that with the healthy fats people in the Mediterranean consume, that allows your body to slowly decrease the amount of unhealthy triglycerides you are consuming and improve overall heart health.

Helps you lose weight in a healthy way. If you're looking for a sustainable long-term lifestyle you can follow to lose weight and become overall healthier, the Mediterranean diet is one you can incorporate into your life. This diet isn't about counting calories or starving yourself, but simply adjusting what you eat so it includes more healthy fats instead of processed foods or sugars. Whether you want to tweak the diet to follow a lower protein intake or lower carb, the Mediterranean diet tends to rely on consuming healthy fats. You are eating higher quality protein which is healthier for you like beans, legumes, and fish, instead of relying on a meal full of red meat or dairy. When that healthy eating is coupled with an active lifestyle, that allows for excess weight to burn off. The diet is especially effective at reducing belly fat which can play a role in Type 2 diabetes

---

[1] https://www.ncbi.nlm.nih.gov/pubmed/17058434
[2] http://www.ncbi.nlm.nih.gov/pubmed/23939686

Can help fight cancer. Of course, there's no cure for cancer, but studies have found that the Mediterranean diet provides the most favorable conditions for the body to fight against cancer. A 2013 study at the University of Genoa in Italy found that the Mediterranean diet provides your body with a balanced ratio of omega fatty acids, fiber, and antioxidants found in wine, fruits, vegetables, and olive oil[3]. Providing high amounts of antioxidants is the key in fighting cancer cells and stopping further cell mutation. A study at the Mayo Clinic found that out of 800 people whose colonoscopies were studied, those with advanced colon polyps reported they ate red meat more frequently and their diet did not correspond to foods on the Mediterranean diet[4]. The World Cancer Research Fund reports that eating at least 90 grams of whole grains a day can reduce your risk of colon cancer by almost 20%[5]. That's because the fiber in whole grains prevents any mutations from developing in your digestive tract and keeps your bowel movement regular. With the Mediterranean diet, you are solely trying to eat whole grains which are much healthier for you. Diet only goes so far, of course, and you should get screened regularly at your annual doctor's appointments for any health concerns.

Protects cognitive health. Following the Mediterranean diet and lifestyle could be key in protecting yourself from future neurodegenerative diseases like Parkinson's, dementia, or Alzheimer's. The healthy fats that the Mediterranean diet is full of are known to fight age-related cognitive decline, along with the anti-inflammatory protection that fresh fruits

---

[3] https://www.ncbi.nlm.nih.gov/pubmed/22644232

[4] https://www.mayoclinic.org/diseases-conditions/colon-polyps/symptoms-causes/syc-20352875
[5] https://www.wcrf.org/sites/default/files/CUP%20Colorectal%20Report_2017_Digital.pdf

and vegetables provide. The Taub Institute for Research in Alzheimer's Disease found that the more strictly the individuals in their test group followed the Mediterranean diet, the lower their risk was for developing Alzheimer's disease[6]. Doctors have always encouraged seniors and patients at risk for neurodegenerative diseases to adopt healthier eating habits to possibly delay their symptoms or onset of dementia. Following a Mediterranean diet can improve your memory, mental acuity, and attention span as it protects your nerve cells from deteriorating with age.

Can increase your life span! A famous study called the Lyon Diet Heart Study studied a group of test individuals who had heart attacks between 1988 and 1992. They were counseled to follow a traditional post-heart attack diet or the Mediterranean diet. When a follow-up study was conducted after 4 years, the results found that the people following the Mediterranean diet had 70% less chance of heart disease[7]. They also experienced a nearly 50% lower risk of death than the standard low-fat diet. It seems that the combination of fresh fruits and vegetables and healthy fat sources like beans, nuts, and fish is a winning combination to extend the human lifespan. Olive oil and nuts contain monounsaturated fats which also contain heart healthy benefits like reducing inflammatory diseases, protecting against cognitive decline and neurodegenerative diseases like Alzheimer's, and lower levels of heart disease, cancer, and depression.

---

[6] https://www.ncbi.nlm.nih.gov/pubmed/16622828

[7] https://www.ahajournals.org/doi/pdf/10.1161/01.cir.99.6.779

Fights depression. A 2018 study published in the Journal of Molecular Psychiatry which found evidence to believe that healthy dietary choices, such as following the Mediterranean diet, can help reduce the risk of depression[8]. That's because it has been shown that the risk decreased when people followed diets that included a variety of anti-inflammatory diseases. Inflammation is often named as one of the root causes of many psychiatric and mental conditions such as obsessive-compulsive disorder, depression, anxiety, and schizophrenia. The study compared a handful of diets including the Mediterranean diet, the Dietary Inflammatory Index, the DASH (Dietary Approaches to Stop Hypertension) diet, and the HEI (Healthy Eating Index), and found that the Mediterranean diet had the most significant decrease in depression in patients.

Protects against Type 2 diabetes. The types of food that the Mediterranean diet encourages such as whole grains, beans, and legumes, contain high amounts of fiber which help to slow digestion and prevent frequent spikes in blood sugar levels. That means you feel full longer without needing a snack. When you are eating, you are limiting yourself to less processed foods and the fat you are obtaining are mostly from olive oil, nuts, and healthy meats. That means the amount of carbohydrates you're intaking is less. It's not a "low carb" diet, but it's one that still reduces the amount of carbohydrates you're intaking so less carbs are converted to glucose. In fact, a 2011 study in Spain found that after a 4-year research study, participants assigned to a Mediterranean style diet had more than 50% less risk of developing Type 2 diabetes[9]! That's compared to the other study group that followed

---

[8] http://www.psychiatrictimes.com/special-reports/introduction-inflammation-connection

[9] http://care.diabetesjournals.org/content/34/1/14

a low-fat diet. The Mediterranean diet encourages meals seasoned with healthy spices, and encourages you to fill your dessert with fruit instead of baked goods that contain sugar.

It is also important to note that in many studies, participants on the Mediterranean diet tended to lose on average more weight than participants on other low carb or low-fat diets. Due to this weight loss, you can reduce your risk of diabetes, and maybe even delay needing medication.

Can reduce risk of erectile dysfunction in men. ED, or erectile dysfunction, is a common side effect of cardiovascular disease. As the blood vessels are blocked with unhealthy plaque, the smaller vessels leading towards the male genitalia are unable to respond like they used to. But research shows the Mediterranean diet can help with this! A study in Italy found tested a group of nearly 70 men by putting half on a control diet and half on a Mediterranean diet. After two years of study, more than one-third of the men who followed the Mediterranean diet strictly regained normal sexual functioning. Though there's no exact reason for this, it's believed that the fiber and healthy antioxidants in fresh fruits and vegetables can promote blood flow throughout the body.

Improves sight. Since the Mediterranean diet is full of fruits, vegetables, and regular servings of fish, it can be great in protecting your sight. According to the American Academy of Ophthalmology, eye health is protected by eating antioxidants which are found in fresh plant products[10]. Fish is also high in omega 3 fatty acids which is critical to sight health. Just having 1 serving of fish in a week can lower the risk of developing eye damage which occurs commonly in people over the age of 50. With the Mediterranean diet, you're incorporating fish in your diet more than 3 times a week! The seeds and nuts you're eating as snacks also contain fatty acids that protect the retinas from cellular damage with age.

Your kidney function improves. Your kidneys are constantly working throughout the day to filter waste and liquid from your body while still maintaining your blood pressure. But chronic kidney disease can affect more than 30 million Americans a year. A 2014 study in the *Clinical Journal of American Society of Nephrology* found that following the Mediterranean diet may decrease the chances of having chronic kidney disease by almost 50%[11]. This could be attributed to clean and healthy food choices that the Mediterranean diet requires, with less processed food and red meat. Fish, fresh fruits and vegetables, and nuts are known to lower inflammation in the body, which can be a culprit of kidney disease.

Can improve your gut health. A 2018 study published in *Nutrition Gastrointestinal Sciences* found that the Mediterranean diet can improve the quantity of good bacteria in your gut due to its mostly plant-based diet[12]. A research study was conducted on 20 non-human primates where they followed either a Western diet or a Mediterranean diet for 30 months. After studying rectal-content samples, it was found that the Mediterranean diet followers had higher gut bacteria diversity and almost 10% more good bacteria compared to

---

[10] https://nei.nih.gov/health/maculardegen/armd_facts

[11] https://cjasn.asnjournals.org/content/9/11/1868
[12] https://www.frontiersin.org/articles/10.3389/fnut.2018.00028/full

just 0.5% for the meat-focused diet followers. These probiotic bacteria are very helpful in the gut and thus, keeps the body steady. If there is no proper balance of bacteria, the body can suffer gastrointestinal issues.

Keeps your bones strong as you get older. In many demographics, women tend to lose bone density and muscle mass as they age and go through menopause. Researchers aimed to find out whether this was true regarding those women who followed the Mediterranean diet more strictly. More than 100 Brazilian women who were on average 55 years old were studied including factors like their calcium mineral density, body fat, and skeletal mass. After the study was completed, it was found that the women who followed diets like the Mediterranean diet, had higher bone density and muscle mass than women who followed a diet with more red meat. Lead researchers at the **Universidade Federal do Rio Grande do Sul in Brazil** where the study was conducted, found that the Mediterranean diet could be a useful lifestyle change for women to conserve bone mass if they are going through menopause or have osteoporosis. It is important to note that this lifestyle should be followed before the body starts menopause. It is not a "quick fix" solution. Any senior who is agile and flexible in their old age will tell you that they have consistently eaten a healthy diet full of fruits, vegetables, and less red meat and unhealthy fats.

Keeps your skin healthy. A diet rich in antioxidants found in fresh fruits and vegetables like the Mediterranean diet helps to keep your skin at its healthiest. That means a healthy grow, strong elasticity, and preventing common skin conditions like eczema, acne, or rosacea. One of the worst foods for your skin is actually sugar which can cause acne breakouts and destroy the healthy collagen in your skin. By following the Mediterranean diet, participants cut out extra sugar and instead rely on healthy fruits with natural sugars. A study even found that people with higher blood sugar levels who battled with spikes in their glucose levels were considered "older looking" based on the appearance of their skin compared to people with low blood sugar levels. Eating a balanced diet full of healthy vitamins and minerals is what keeps your skin healthy and that's exactly what the Mediterranean diet provides!

Protect the body from stress and aging. Studies show that the Mediterranean diet reduces inflammation in the body and also helps to protect the body against oxidative stress. Aging in our cells is common but the healthier our cells remain, the more active we will be for longer. The Mediterranean diet follows a lot of recommendations that are noted for anti-aging benefits such as limiting the intake of red meat, having a small amount of wine with meals, and limiting processed or unhealthy sugars. These dietary changes are a part of the Mediterranean diet, which means you can feel the benefits of healthy skin, more energy, and longevity of your cells, especially the nerve cells, to keep your brain active and functioning at top mental acuity.

Chapter 4: How to Lose Weight on the Mediterranean Diet

A lot of people think when they start a new diet, it will mean a quick and easy weight loss method. But the Mediterranean diet is not meant to be a traditional diet, in the sense that you do it for a little while, lose the weight, then go back to your old habits. This method is a true lifestyle change to embark on a healthy eating journey. Making those significant changes will help you achieve your weight loss goals and also gain the other health benefits we mentioned in Chapter 3. You will still get to eat a variety of delicious foods, but you are simply changing what you eat to fit this lifestyle. With this method, it is relatively easy, in the sense that you don't have to count calories or tabulate your macronutrients for the day. But in order to see progressive results, you will have to make changes.

How can you begin the steps to embark on this diet and see positive results? Here are some tips on how you can begin.

Change Your Lifestyle: The Mediterranean diet is about making changes in your lifestyle to see beneficial long-term results. That means changing your diet, decreasing your portions sizes, and incorporating regular exercise into your routine. By being consistent with these changes, you will lose weight and be able to keep the weight off compared to other "quick fix" diets that offer only a temporary solution. What are some steps to begin this journey?

- Quit other diets you may be on. If you're convinced that the Mediterranean diet is right for you, commit to it in order to see the long-term results. If you see it as a quick solution, or you have other diet fads you fall suspect to, then you won't be able to truly follow this lifestyle.

- Set realistic goals. You have to be able to set goals and achieve them so you can make progress. This means that that you are ready to do things like cleaning your pantry of processed foods and unhealthy oils, and incorporating more fish into your diet. Also, this includes trying new Mediterranean recipes so you become familiar with the ingredients, and that you aren't continuing to eat dinners full of red meat. You want to steadily make progress so you can see measurable goals such as losing a couple pounds or a decrease in your cholesterol numbers. Achieving these small goals will properly motivate you to continue your journey and see what other health benefits you could gain.

- Stick to the changes. Use these goals as a way to build upon the diet. You don't want to end up going backward! Remind yourself how far you've come and how you want to continue to stay healthy to avoid the risk of heart disease, diabetes, or other health conditions that you may be battling or have a family history of.

Be Aware of Your Calories: If you've tried a variety of diets before settling on the Mediterranean one, then you're familiar with the concept of counting calories and staying calorie deficit. That is a crucial concept of losing weight. How fast your body burns calories daily depends on your individual metabolic rate. Factors such as gender, body frame, age, genetics, and physical fitness level all play a role in how fast your body will burn calories. In order to lose weight, you must be burning more calories than you consume. That means if you lead a sedentary lifestyle, you're not burning as much as you're taking in which will not allow your body to burn excess fat. You must be calorie deficit.

With the Mediterranean diet, it's not necessary that you count the calories you're eating daily, but it's still important that you are aware of what you are eating and how big your portion is. By making small lifestyle changes, you can be more attentive to your caloric intake and compare it to how your weight loss goals are going. What are some things to be aware of?

- Be aware of your portion size. Paying attention to what size portion you are eating is a lot easier than having to count calories every meal. Often, in the United States, the portion sizes for a meal are a lot bigger. An entree can take up nearly all of your plate! Remember that portion sizes in the Mediterranean tend to be different and people focus more on the quality of the food they are eating rather than quantity. This isn't to say that you shouldn't eat enough or should starve yourself, but simply be aware of how big your portion size is, and if you can get away with eating a few bites less.

- Eat more filling foods. One of the things about the Mediterranean diet is that it allows you have to more filling foods that consist of fewer calories. That sounds too good to be true, doesn't it? But by eating more low-calorie vegetables, like broccoli, brussels sprouts, or cabbage, you can eat a bigger quantity compared to very high-calorie foods like red meat. These vegetables and fruits often contain a lot of fiber which allows you to feel fuller longer. Hopefully, you will be less tempted to reach for a snack right after your meal. Less snacking means less calories!

- Keep an eye on your fat calories. Even though the Mediterranean diet recommends healthy fats such as olive oil and nuts, you still want to be aware of how much of those fats you are including in your diet. If you are unknowingly consuming too much fat, even if they are healthy fats, you won't see weight loss. Remember, don't use 2 tablespoons of oil when 1 will do! Though it's important you switch from trans fats like butter or margarine, you should still remain aware of how much of your daily calorie intake is coming from fats.

- Get moving! Exercise is important in the Mediterranean diet because it reflects how the people of the Mediterranean live(d). The people whose diet we are trying to emulate lived a very active lifestyle well into their old age. You'll never truly achieve weight loss until you burn some of the calories you're eating! Otherwise, they will simply be stored away as extra fat reserves. Exercise lets you burn those calories and has lots of other side effects like managing stress, releasing endorphins to improve your mood, increasing your energy level, and helping you have a better night's sleep. Whether it's a bike ride around your neighborhood or half an hour at the gym, incorporate physical activity into your week more regularly so you can see weight loss results.

Control Your Cravings (Don't Let Them Control You!): Food cravings are a natural part of dieting. Whether they're actual physical reactions in the body or a psychological reaction to being deprived of certain foods, it is still important that you learn to control your cravings and distract yourself so you aren't tempted to cheat on your new Mediterranean lifestyle! There is no simple answer to solving those cravings, but it's still important that you try different things to control them and suppress your appetite.

- Try not to skip meals. Have a meal or snack every 4 to 5 hours. If you end up skipping a meal or waiting until you are extremely hungry, science proves that you will end up eating an excessive amount of calories. To prevent overeating, set your meal times and follow that routine no matter how busy your day. Plan your meals in advance or meal prep so you know what you have to cook and aren't tempted to grab an easy, non-Mediterranean diet meal!

- Load up on fiber. As we mentioned in the previous section, eating fiber-rich foods will allow you to feel full longer. You don't have to eat these foods all at once, but try and incorporate vegetables or whole grains in your meals as a side or as a snack. Whether it's a quick chopped salad, some saluted veggies or whole grain cereal, spread these snacks throughout your day so you will stay full until your next meal. This will keep you less likely to reach for unhealthy snacks.

- Eat protein-rich foods. Though you still want to avoid filling your diet with red meat, you can incorporate other protein-rich foods that will slow down your digestion and keep you full. That includes food like lentils, beans, fish, eggs, and nuts. Try having a handful of raw nuts as a snack, or make a quick lentil soup. These foods tend to be low in calories but still have a high protein content so you feel like you've had a filling meal.

- Manage the stress in your life. Stress hormones will disrupt your health no matter how strictly you are trying to follow a new diet! Cortisol is the natural stress hormone the body releases when it feels stressed. Too much cortisol in the bloodstream can cause mood swings, weight gain, irritability and trouble sleeping. Be aware of the stressful factors in your life and do your best to control your reaction to them. You can try incorporating a routine of meditation, deep breathing, or a spa day to help yourself relax. You may want to try getting regular exercise, enough sleep, and staying hydrated to help you feel more relaxed, and able to cope with any upcoming stress. Getting enough rest is also important so be sure you have a bedtime routine that includes no screens, and relaxing or meditating before bed to help you have a good night's rest. With the Mediterranean diet, you should be having less artificial sugar which means your blood sugar levels will be stable enough to help you remain calm before bed.

Remember, how far you want to see long-term results depends on how steadfast you are about following the diet. If you see it as only a temporary method, you may be disappointed to see weight gain. If you embrace it as a true lifestyle change, you could see some of the health benefits we described and keep weight off in the long-term.

Chapter 5: The Mediterranean Diet Pyramid & Your Shopping List

The Mediterranean Diet Pyramid is a nutritional guide that was developed by the World Health Organization in 1993. It was also worked on by the Harvard School of Public Health, and the Oldways Preservation Trust. It is a visual tool that summarizes the Mediterranean Diet's suggested pattern of eating and gives a guide to how frequently specific tools should be eaten. This allows you to have a breakdown of healthy eating habits and not overfill yourself with too many calories.

How is the pyramid laid out? Let's go over each tier.

Olive oil, fruits, vegetables, whole grains, legumes, beans, nuts & seeds, spices & herbs: These are the types of food that form the base of the Mediterranean pyramid. You'll notice that these are mostly from plant sources. You should try and include a few variations of these items into each meal you eat. Olive oil should be the main fat you use in your cooking and your dishes, so replace any other butter or cooking oil you used to use. Generous uses of herbs and spices are also encouraged to season your food and add flavor as an alternative to salt. If you don't have access to fresh herbs, you can buy the dried version. Always be sure to read the nutrition labels to ensure there are no other ingredients mixed with the herbs. Fresh ginger and garlic are also great flavor enhancers for your meals. They can be easily stored in the freezer.

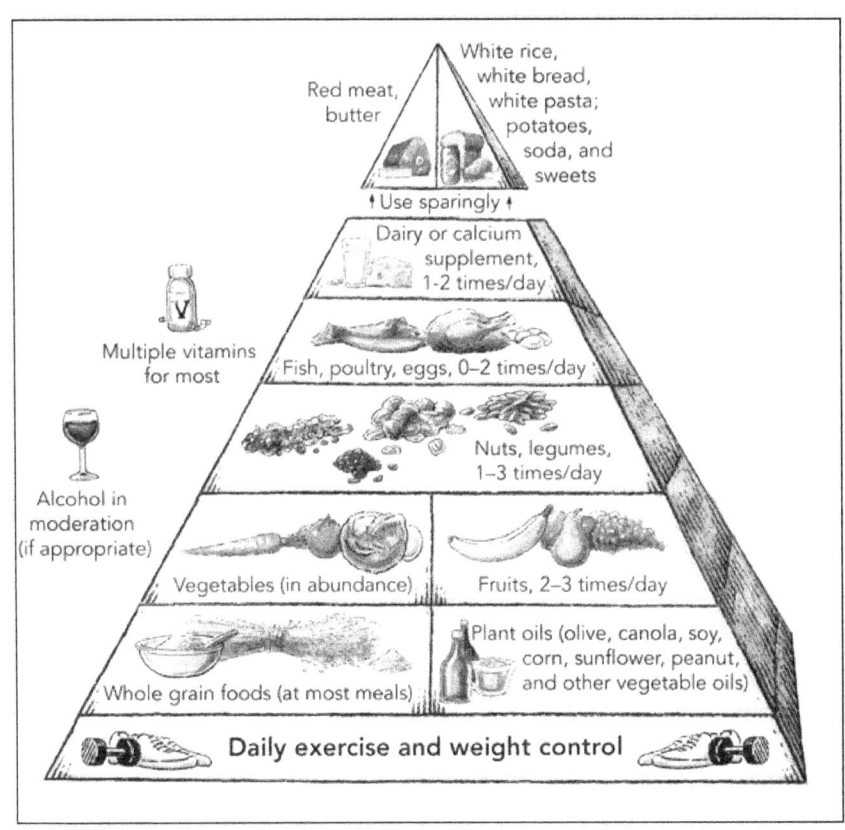

Fish & seafood: These are important staples of the Mediterranean diet that should be consumed often as a protein source. You want to try and include these in your diet at least two times a week. Try new varieties of fish, either frozen or fresh. Also incorporate seafood like mussels, crab, and shrimp into your diet. Canned tuna is also great to include on sandwiches or toss in a salad with fresh vegetables.

Cheese, yogurt, eggs & poultry: These ingredients should be consumed in more moderate amounts when on the Mediterranean diet. Depending on the food, they should be used sparingly throughout the week. Keep in mind that if you are using eggs in baking or cooking, those will also be counted in your weekly limit. You want to stick to more healthy cheese like Parmesan, ricotta, or feta that you can add as a topping or garnish on your dishes.

Red meat & sweets: These items are going to be consumed less frequently when on the Mediterranean diet. If you are eating them, you want to be sure it is only in small quantities and prefer lean meat versions with less fat. Most studies recommend a maximum of 12 to 16 ounces per month. You can still have red meat on occasion to add some variety to your diet, but you want to reduce how often you have it. That's because of all the health concerns that come with sugar and red meat. The Mediterranean diet is working to improve cardiovascular health and reduce blood pressure, while red meat tends to be dangerous in terms of cardiac health. The residents of Greece ate very little red meat and instead had fish or seafood as their main source of protein.

Water: The Mediterranean diet encourages you to be hydrated so that means drinking more than your daily intake of water. Depending on how active you are and what climate you are in, your intake can vary. The Institute of Medicine recommends a total of 9 cups each day for women, and 13 cups for men. If a woman is pregnant or breastfeeding, that number should be increased.

Wine: Moderate consumption of wine with meals is encouraged on the Mediterranean diet. Studies have shown that moderate consumption of alcohol can reduce the risk of heart disease. That can mean about 1 glass per day for women. Men tend to have higher body mass so they can consume 1 to 2 glasses. Please keep in mind what your doctor would recommend regarding wine consumption based on your individual health and family history.

Your Mediterranean Diet Shopping List

To make it easier for you, we have suggestions of what exactly to include on your shopping list to follow the Mediterranean diet! We'll let you know what you need to include and what you need to leave out.

Include:

- *Extra virgin and virgin olive oils*: These are going to be the least processed and refined versions of olive oil on the market. They will contain the highest level of plant compounds called "phenols" that act as antioxidants in the body. Not all olive oils are created equally so be sure you're checking for the "extra virgin" label and using a highly recommended brand that you trust. It might be a little pricier than the oil you used before, but it's well worth it when you're aware of the health benefits you will gain! This will be your go-to when it comes to cooking, frying, seasoning, and as the base of your salad dressings. Remember, less is more!

- *Fish & Seafood*: Whether it's mackerel, trout, sardines, tuna, salmon, or tilapia, fish is going to be a staple for you on the Mediterranean diet! These types of fatty fish are going to be rich sources of omega 3 fatty acids throughout the week. Be sure to experiment with new types so you don't get tired of the same one! You can even use canned fish like sardines or anchovies because cured fish was very common in Greece. Try and look for the low sodium versions though to avoid excess salt intake. Don't forget shrimp, crab, or mussels so you can expand your seafood palate!

- *Vegetables:* You have pretty much free rein with vegetables though if you can stick to low-calorie ones, that's even better for your weight loss goals. Vegetables like zucchini, mushrooms, cabbage, cauliflower, bell pepper, and spinach are low in calories but are still very filling and high in fiber. Try new vegetables and eating them in different ways like a green smoothie or different salad combination so you don't get bored. Try to buy in season items so you can save yourself some money!

- *Fruits:* Fruits are encouraged and are great as a substitute healthy dessert to treat yourself to. Figs and pomegranates are native to the Mediterranean area, but any fruit will do! Be sure to include a variety of colorful fruits and vegetables which allow you to have a diverse range of essential vitamins and minerals. Be mindful of how much fruit you are eating though, because you don't want to have an excess number of calories or natural sugars which will interfere with your weight loss. If you are diabetic, try and consume fruits that are low on the glycemic index such as oranges, apples, grapefruits, pears, or plums.

- *Legumes & beans:* These are a great hidden source of protein which often get overlooked in the West in favor of red meat or poultry items. Thankfully, the Mediterranean diet urges you to try different variations of protein sources! Whether it's black beans, kidney beans, chickpeas, or lentils, these are great to experiment with. Don't forget hummus! These are packed with fiber as well, so they allow you to feel full for longer. Be sure you drink plenty of water to avoid constipation!

- *Whole grain breads and cereal:* Whether it's rice, barley, oats, leek rice, quinoa, whole grain pasta, or whole grain bread, you want to be sure you are focused on whole grains that are healthier rather than refined or processed grains. Same goes with cereal. Be sure you read the label and ensure the product is made from whole grain starches and are not processed into refined products. Ezekiel bread is a whole grain bread made with no sugar. One slice is packed with fiber and contains only 80 calories! The trick with whole grains is that you can eat a smaller portion than you would with refined wheat products, but stay full longer. These are also low on the glycemic index scale which makes them safe for diabetes patients.

- *Nuts & seeds*: This includes items like cashews, pistachios, walnuts, sunflower seeds, pine nuts, flax seeds, almonds, and other nuts which may be your favorites. Keep these as a healthy snack throughout the day, but be sure to avoid the chocolate-covered or salted versions which are unhealthy. You want to stick to the raw nuts. Chia seeds are also tiny but powerful! In just 2 tablespoons, you can have 11 grams of fiber! These are great to add to a smoothie or as a topping on oatmeal or cereal to fill you up. The great thing is they're almost flavorless so anyone can incorporate them into their meals!

- *Low-fat dairy*: If you are used to dairy products in your diet, you don't have to cut them out entirely but it's better you switch to low-fat versions. Use fat-free yogurt or low-fat cheese, and switch to skim or reduced fat milk. On the Mediterranean diet you want most of your dairy calories to come from healthy cheeses like feta, brie, Greek yogurt, or Parmesan.

- *Herbs & spices:* These are great to season your food with and add a great distinct flavor other than salt. You can try using fresh herbs like rosemary and parsley though they may not last as long in your refrigerator. You can always start a windowsill herb garden which are easy to maintain! If not, don't be intimidated and feel free to use dried herbs from the spice aisle. Experiment with new flavors that will enhance your flavor profile. Fresh garlic and ginger are also great flavor enhancers and considered essentials of Greek and Mediterranean cuisine. They have multiple health benefits and pack your meals with flavor.

Exclude:

- *Red meat*: As we mentioned, you want to go light on red meat portions when you are shopping for your Mediterranean diet. If you do want to get a few portions, be sure they're smaller sized and lean meat cuts that have less fat. Try to only have it once a week and keep an eye on your portion size. Also, avoid high-fat processed meats like pre-made sausages or hot dogs which are loaded with preservatives and high in sodium. These tend to cause inflammation in the body.

- *Poultry*: Again, you want to use poultry in your diet less often than you would on other diets. More lean cuts with less fat can be used now and then as long as you have smaller portions. For the most part, try and substitute your red meat and poultry meals with fish or seafood, although it's okay to have them once in a while during the week. Turkey or duck would be a healthier alternative to chicken because they contain less fat.

- *Refined grains*: These include things like bagels, cereal, or white bread that we might previously consider staples in our diet. But these should be excluded from your shopping list unless you have verified that the cereals, pasta, or bread are whole grain certified products.

- *Sugars:* That means skipping things like candy, chocolate, ice cream, sugary juices, and sodas! Instead, try and treat yourself to berries or fruit as a sweet treat, or enhance your water with lemon or mint leaves for more flavor. Get used to the habit of having natural sugars in fruit as a dessert instead of wanting unhealthy baked goods.

- *Trans or saturated fats*: Exclude things like butter or margarine which contain unhealthy saturated fats. You want to substitute any unhealthy oils like canola oil or vegetable oil with the healthier option of extra virgin olive oil. You want to use this in your cooking, frying, and as the main component of your vinaigrettes.

- *Highly processed foods*: These should be avoided on the Mediterranean diet. The rule of thumb should be if it comes in a box, you can't have it! That's because food that tends to be marked as "low-fat" or "diet friendly" is actually very processed and unhealthy for you. Instead of eating those empty calories, focus on what you can eat as a filling snack like some of the items we mentioned above.

Chapter 6: 14-Day Mediterranean Meal Plan
(with Snack Ideas!)

WEEK 1

MONDAY

Breakfast: Avocado Egg Breakfast Sandwich

Prep Time: 3-4 minutes

Total Time: 10-12 minutes

Nutritional Facts: 2 servings total (302 calories, 28 grams carbs, 10 grams fiber, 12 grams protein, 18 grams fat)

Ingredients:

1 avocado peeled and cut into slices

1 hardboiled egg, sliced

1 teaspoon olive oil

4 slices whole wheat bread, toasted

8-10 asparagus spears, steamed

1 teaspoon Dijon mustard

salt and pepper to taste

Directions:

On two bread slices, spread the mustard. On the other two slices, arrange the avocado. Top with asparagus and egg slices. Season your sandwich and brush with olive oil. You should be able to make 2 sandwiches.

Lunch: Vegetable and Feta Salad

Prep Time: 15-18 minutes

Total Time: 35-40 minutes

Nutritional Facts: 2 servings total (350 calories per serving, 32 grams fat, 13 grams carbs, 6 grams protein)

Ingredients:

1 large cucumber

a pinch of salt & black pepper

.5 cup feta cheese, diced

.5 red onion

1-2 tablespoons olive oil

.5 bell pepper

.25 cup pitted black olives

.25 cup pitted green olives

2 tablespoon minced fresh oregano

1 cup cherry tomatoes

2-3 tablespoons red wine vinegar

Directions:

Wash all your vegetables first. Peel your cucumber if you like it without the peel. Cut into half, then quarter pieces before slicing into about .5" pieces. Toss with some salt and let sit in a bowl for 10 to 15 minutes before you rinse and drain them. Slice your cherry tomatoes in half, and chop your onion, bell pepper and olives to the size you wish. Combine your vegetables in a bowl with half of the minced oregano. Sprinkle in the red wine vinegar, season to taste, and toss. Add the olive oil and add the feta cheese. Refrigerate for about 30 minutes and sprinkle with the rest of the fresh oregano before eating.

Dinner: Rosemary and Walnut Crusted Salmon

Prep Time: 13-15 minutes

Total Time: 35-38 minutes

Nutritional Facts: 4 servings total (222 calories per serving, 12 grams fat, 0 grams fiber, 4 grams carbs, 24 grams protein)

Ingredients:

.5 teaspoon kosher salt

1 tablespoon mustard

2 teaspoons lemon juice

3 teaspoons olive oil

.5 teaspoon crushed red pepper

4 tablespoons bread crumbs

.5 teaspoon lemon zest

1 clove minced garlic

4 tablespoons chopped walnuts

1 1-pound salmon fillet, divided into 4 portions

1 teaspoon fresh rosemary, roughly chopped

olive oil cooking spray

Directions:

First, set your oven to 425 degrees F. Combine the mustard, garlic, lemon juice, rosemary, lemon zest, salt, and pepper in a bowl. Combine the bread crumbs, walnuts, and olive oil to another bowl. Place your salmon on your lined baking sheet and spread the marinade over the fish. Then coat the bread mixture on top to seal it in. You can spray with your olive oil cooking spray at this point to lock in the moisture. Bake uncovered for 8-12 minutes. Your fish should be lightly golden brown and flaky. It will be less time if your filet is thinner.

TUESDAY

Breakfast: Almond Date Smoothies

Prep Time: 3-4 minutes

Total Time: 11-13 minutes

Nutritional Facts: 2 servings total (423 calories per serving, 82 grams carbs, 10 grams fiber, 6 grams protein, 1 gram fat)

Ingredients:

1 tablespoon agave nectar or honey

1 banana

2 tablespoons almond butter

a handful of ice

.5 cup dates, pitted

1 cup unsweetened almond milk

Directions:

Pour the almond milk in a bowl and let the dates soak in the milk. Allow the dates to chill for 10 minutes. In a blender, combine the milk, dates, banana, and almond butter. Add the honey if you prefer a sweeter taste. Add ice and blend until smooth.

Lunch: Meat, Cheese & Melon Plate

Prep Time: 11-13 minutes

Total Time: 22-25 minutes

Nutritional Facts: 2 servings total (1 plate per serving, 546 calories per serving, 32 grams fat, 42 grams carbs, 24 grams protein)

Ingredients:

1 cup cantaloupe, cubed

.5 cup cherry tomatoes, halved

.5 cup unsalted hazelnuts

6 .25" thick whole wheat bread slices

10 fresh Mozzarella cheese balls

6 slices prosciutto, halved

Directions:

Divide all the items equally between two plates and serve.

Dinner: Greek Fish Tacos

Prep time: 14-16 minutes

Total time: 25-35 minutes

Nutritional Facts: 8 servings total (248 calories per serving, 8 grams fat, 13 grams protein, 6 grams carbs)

Ingredients:

1 cup cherry tomatoes, halved

.5 cup feta cheese, crumbled

tzatziki sauce for topping

2 cups shredded cabbage

1 cup pitted olives

8 small soft whole wheat tortillas

salt and pepper to taste

2 tablespoons olive oil

1 pound firm fish such as cod, tilapia, catfish, mahi mahi

Directions:

First, season your fish. In a medium pan on medium heat, add the olive oil and cook the fish for 4-6 minutes on each side until cooked through. Remove from heat and use a fork and knife to cut into bite-sized pieces. Assemble your tacos in the flour tortillas by layering the cabbage, tomatoes, olives, fish, and feta cheese. Add the tzatziki sauce as a topping.

WEDNESDAY

Breakfast: Overnight Oats w/ Fruit

Prep Time: 4-5 minutes

Total Time: 3 to 12 hours depending

Nutritional Facts: 4 servings total (530 calories per serving, 18 grams fat, 78 grams carbs, 10 grams fiber, 18 grams protein)

Ingredients:

2 cups regular rolled oats

1.5 teaspoon ground cinnamon

.75 cup chopped raw nuts of your choice

1 cup milk

.25 cup honey or agave nectar

1 6-ounce container of yogurt

1 cup berries of your choice

1 green apple, seeded, sliced

Directions:

Have 4 mason jars that you can prepare. Divide the oats into .5 cup servings in each mason jar. In a bowl, combine the cinnamon, milk, and honey. Divide by pouring a section into each mason jar of oats. Cover and chill overnight or for a few hours until oats are soft. Top with nuts and fruit.

Lunch: Feta Garbanzo Bean Salad

Prep Time: 12-14 minutes

Total Time: 18-20 minutes

Nutritional Facts: 4 servings total (2 cups salad per serving, 275 calories, 17 grams fat, 8 grams fiber, 11 grams protein, 22 grams carbs,)

Ingredients:

.25 cup fresh parsley, chopped

1 can (~14 ounces) garbanzo beans

.5 cup pitted olives, sliced

.5 cup onion, sliced

1 tomato, chopped

2-3 tablespoons olive oil

.5 cup feta cheese, crumbled

salt and pepper to taste

3.5 cups salad greens

1 cup cucumber, chopped

Directions:

In a salad bowl, add the vegetables and toss with olive oil. Add seasoning and top with feta cheese.

Dinner: Greek Lemon Chicken Soup

Prep Time: 12-14 minutes

Total Time: 28-32 minutes

Nutritional Facts: 4 servings total (451 calories per serving, 15 grams fat, 40 grams carbs, 30 grams protein)

Ingredients:

1 cup orzo

.25 cup fresh lemon juice

1 cup cooked and shredded chicken breast

3 eggs

4 cups chicken stock

1 teaspoon olive oil

salt and pepper to taste

Directions:

In a pot, add the chicken stock. When it comes to a boil, add the olive oil and orzo. Cook the orzo until it has become firm. While the orzo is cooking, whisk together the eggs and lemon juice. When the orzo is done, ladle out 1 cup of the chicken broth. Slowly add a tablespoon of broth to the egg mixture at a time, and whisk so it combines. Then add it back to the pot of chicken broth. You want to add your shredded chicken now and salt and pepper to your taste. Stir until the soup has thickened.

THURSDAY

Breakfast: White Egg Omelet

Prep Time: 6-8 minutes

Total Time: 10-12 minutes

Nutritional Facts: 1 serving total (72 calories per serving, 2 grams fat, 1 gram carbs, 0 grams fiber, 11 grams protein)

Ingredients:

a dash of black pepper

.5 teaspoon olive oil

3 egg whites (it can be 2 egg whites + 1 whole egg, or .5 cup egg white product)

1 teaspoon fresh cut herbs of your choice

Directions:

In a small bowl, add your egg whites and sprinkle with black pepper. Add in any fresh herb of your choice like parsley or rosemary. Beat with a fork until combined. In a small skillet on medium heat, add the olive oil and pour in your egg mixture. You will want to cook until the edges crinkle and the mixture is set and cooked through. Use a spatula to flip and cook the other side. Remove from heat.

Lunch: Spanish Garlic Shrimp

Prep Time: 12-14 minutes

Total Time: 17-19 minutes

Nutritional Facts: 4 servings total (250 calories per total, 17.9 grams fat, 3.9 grams carbs, 16 grams protein, .5 grams fiber)

Ingredients:

2 tablespoons lemon juice

.75 teaspoon paprika

.25 teaspoon chili flakes

1 pound large shrimp, peeled

.25 cup olive oil

2-3 tablespoons parsley, chopped

3 cloves garlic, minced

salt and pepper to taste

2 tablespoons dry sherry

Directions:

In a large skillet on medium heat, first add olive oil and garlic. Once garlic is fragrant, add the shrimp to the pan. Add salt, pepper, chili flakes, and paprika for seasoning. Cook your shrimp on both sides. Add your sherry and lemon juice to the pan and stir until the liquid has reduced. Sprinkle parsley on top as garnishing.

Dinner: Bruschetta Steak

Prep Time: 16-18 minutes

Total Time: 26-30 minutes

Nutritional Facts: 4 servings total (1 steak piece w/ .5 cup salad, 280 calories per serving, 20 grams fat, 5 grams carbs, 20 grams protein)

Ingredients:

2 tablespoons fresh basil, chopped

3 clove garlic, minced

3 tomatoes, roughly chopped

2 tablespoons fresh parsley, chopped

salt and pepper to taste

3 tablespoons olive oil

1 1-pound sirloin steak, divided into 4 pieces

1 tablespoon fresh oregano, chopped

.25 cup Parmesan cheese, grated

Directions:

Combine the tomatoes, basil, parsley, oregano, garlic. Add the olive oil, pepper, and salt. Season the beef with your spices. Grill the meat over medium heat or broil until cooked through. Garnish with your salad and the grated cheese.

FRIDAY

Breakfast: Mediterranean Scrambled Eggs

Prep Time: 3-4 minutes

Total Time: 10-12 minutes

Nutritional Facts: 2 servings total (242 calories per serving, 3 grams fiber, 17 grams fat, 13 grams carbs)

Ingredients:

salt and pepper to taste

2 spring onions, sliced

6-8 cherry tomatoes, halved

2 tablespoons black olives, sliced

4 eggs

.25 teaspoon dried oregano

1-2 tablespoons olive oil

.5 teaspoon parsley, chopped

1 yellow pepper, diced

Directions:

In a pan on medium heat, add the olive oil, pepper and chopped spring onions. Lightly fry until the vegetables become soft. Add the tomatoes and olives. Add your eggs to the pan and scramble using a spatula. At this point, season your eggs and garnish with the fresh herbs. Keep stirring until the eggs are fully cooked. Remove from heat.

Lunch: Lentil Garlic Bowls

Prep Time: 16-18 minutes

Total Time: 26-28 minutes

Nutritional Facts: 6 servings total (.75 cup per serving, 287 calories per serving, 4 grams fat, 50 grams carbs, 21 grams protein, 8 grams fiber)

Ingredients:

1 tablespoon olive oil

.5 teaspoon ginger powder

3 cloves garlic, minced

salt and pepper to taste

.5 teaspoon paprika

2 cups dried brown lentils

2 onions, chopped

4 cups water

3 teaspoons lemon juice

.25 cup tomato sauce

.75 cup fat-free Greek yogurt

Directions:

In a large pan on medium heat, add the olive oil and lightly sauté the onions until golden brown. Add garlic and cook until fragrant. Next, add your cups of water along with the lentils. Add your seasonings of salt, pepper, ginger powder, and paprika. Cook until the lentils become tender. Add the tomato sauce and lemon juice. Serve with yogurt.

Dinner: Slow Cooker Mediterranean Chicken

Prep Time: 1-15 minutes

Total Time: 3 to 4.5 hours

Nutritional Facts: 4 servings total (302 calories per serving, 13 grams fat, 6 grams carbs, 2 grams fat, 27 grams protein)

Ingredients:

3-4 cloves garlic, minced

2 onions, chopped

1 cup bell pepper, diced

3 tablespoons lemon juice

1 cup pitted olives

3 tablespoon Italian seasoning

4 medium chicken breasts, boneless, skinless

fresh basil for garnishing

salt and pepper to taste

Directions:

Season the chicken to taste. In a pan on medium heat, cook the chicken until it's no longer raw. Add the chicken pieces to a slow cooker. Add the olives, peppers, and onions to the slow cooker. Mix together the lemon juice, Italian seasoning, and garlic, and pour over the chicken. Depending on how fast you want your meal cooked, you can set your slow cooker for low (4 hours) or high (2 hours). Garnish with fresh basil and serve.

SATURDAY

Breakfast: Mediterranean Keto Low Carb Egg Muffins

Prep Time: 8-10 minutes

Total Time: 20-25 minutes

Nutritional Facts: 6 servings total (1 muffin per serving, 109 calories per serving, 6.3 grams fat, 2 grams carbs, 1.8 grams fiber, 9.2 grams protein)

Ingredients:

2 tablespoons pesto sauce

pinch of salt & pepper

5 eggs

.25 cup feta cheese, crumbled

.5 cup fresh spinach, cut finely

8-10 slices deli ham, thinly sliced

.5 cup bell pepper, sliced

2 tablespoons fresh basil for garnishing

Directions:

Set your oven to 400 degrees F. You can use silicone or paper liners to line your muffin tray. Place at the bottom of each muffin tin with 1.5 pieces of ham. Don't leave any holes. Place a slice of bell pepper. Top with spinach and feta cheese. In a bowl, season the eggs with salt and pepper. Add the egg mixture into 6 muffin tins. Bake until the mixture is set and golden in color, anywhere from 12-16 minutes. Garnish each muffin with pesto sauce, any leftover bell pepper, and fresh basil.

Lunch: *California Quinoa Bowl*

Prep Time: 16-18 minutes

Total Time: 28-30 minutes

Nutritional Facts: 4 servings total (1 cup per serving, 40 grams carbs, 10 grams fat, 6 grams fiber, 14 grams protein)

Ingredients:

1 cup quinoa, rinsed and drained

4 cloves garlic, minced

.75 cup garbanzo beans

1 tomato, chopped

3 tablespoons olive oil

.5 cup feta cheese, crumbled

1 zucchini, chopped

2 cups water

2 tablespoons fresh basil, chopped

.25 cup pitted olives, sliced

Directions:

In a large saucepan on medium heat, add the olive oil first. Stir in the quinoa and garlic until golden brown in color. Next, add the water and zucchini and let the mixture boil. Reduce the liquid by letting it simmer for 15 minutes. Add the remaining ingredients.

Dinner: Greek Turkey Meatball Gyro w/ Tzatziki

Prep Time: 12-14 minutes

Total Time: 22-25 minutes

Nutritional Facts: 4 servings total (1 flatbread + 3 meatballs) (429 calories per serving, 19 grams fat, 39 grams carbs, 27 grams protein, 4 grams fiber)

Ingredients:

4 whole wheat flatbreads

.25 cup red onion, sliced

1 cup diced tomato

.75 cup diced cucumber

Meatballs:

3 tablespoons olive oil

.5 cup red onion, diced

1 tablespoon oregano

1 pound ground turkey

1 cup fresh spinach, chopped

3 cloves garlic, minced

salt and pepper to taste

Tzatziki Sauce:

3 teaspoons lemon juice

.5 teaspoon dry dill

.5 teaspoon garlic powder

salt and black pepper to taste

.5 cup plain Greek yogurt

Directions:

Combine the ground turkey, red onion, salt, fresh spinach, oregano, black pepper, and garlic in a large bowl. It may be easier to mix together with your hands until the meat sticks together. Then form about 1-inch meatballs. You should be able to make about 12 meatballs. In a frying pan, lightly pan fry the meatballs in olive oil for 3-4 minutes until brown. Remove from pan and let excess oil drain on a paper towel. Combine all your Tzatziki sauce ingredients to a bowl and add pepper and salt. To each flatbread, you can add 3 meatballs, the diced tomato, cucumber, and onion vegetables, and top with Tzatziki sauce.

SUNDAY

Breakfast: Mediterranean Breakfast Sandwich

Prep Time: 7-8 minutes

Total Time: 12-14 minutes

Nutritional Facts: 2 servings total (1 sandwich per serving, 247 calories per serving, 12 grams fat, 13 grams protein, 24 grams carbs, 6 grams fiber)

Ingredients:

2 whole grain sandwich thins

salt & black pepper to taste

1 tablespoon fresh rosemary, or half teaspoon dried rosemary herbs

2 tablespoons olive oil

1 tomato, sliced

3 tablespoons feta cheese, sliced

1 cup fresh spinach, chopped

2 eggs

Directions:

Pre-heat your oven to 380 degrees F. Cut the sandwich thins in half and lightly brush both sides with olive oil before placing on a baking sheet. Lightly brown by toasting them in the oven for 2-4 minutes. Add olive oil to a medium sized skillet, then rosemary and eggs. Cook until the whites are set but leave the yolks runny if you prefer it that way. Flip and cook the other side and break the yolks with a spatula. Divide the spinach among the sandwiches and top with tomato, egg, and feta cheese. Sprinkle with salt and pepper. Top with the toasted sandwich halves.

Lunch: Mediterranean Chicken Stir Fry

Prep Time: 16-18 minutes

Total Time: 25 minutes

Nutritional Facts: 4 servings total (1 cup chicken w/ .75 cup rice per serving, 401 calories, 12 grams fat, 38 grams carbs, 29 grams protein)

Ingredients:

salt & pepper to taste

.5 cup pitted green olives, sliced

2 small tomatoes, chopped

1 onion, chopped

1 zucchini, chopped

.25 teaspoon red pepper flakes

3 cloves garlic, minced

1 cup brown rice

2 teaspoons olive oil

1 teaspoon dried oregano

1 teaspoon dried basil

2-3 cups water

1 pound boneless chicken breasts, cubed

Directions:

In a medium pot on the stove, bring the water to a boil before adding the rice and cook as instructed in the packaging. Remove from heat. Add olive oil to a large frying pan or wok. Lightly fry the chicken until it is cooked. Remove from heat. Add the onion into the remaining olive oil. Add the garlic, red pepper, basil, zucchini, oregano. Stir fry until the vegetables become a little softer and season with pepper and salt. Add the cooked chicken, cooked rice, and tomatoes.

Dinner: Grilled Salmon w/ Vegetables

Prep Time: 13-16 minutes

Total Time: 23-26 minutes

Nutritional Facts: 4 servings total (281 calories, 14 grams fat, 10 grams carbs, 30 grams protein, 3 grams fiber, 6 grams sugar)

Ingredients:

1 medium zucchini, diced

2 bell peppers, de-seeded and diced

2 tablespoons olive oil

1 lemon cut into wedges

.25 cup fresh basil, roughly copped

1 teaspoon black pepper

1 1-pound skinless salmon fillet, divided into 4 pieces

2 teaspoons of salt, divided

1 red onion, diced

Directions:

Prepare your grill to medium-high flame. Season the vegetables with olive oil and pepper, and salt. Season your salmon with the remaining salt and some black pepper. Next, arrange your salmon and vegetable pieces skin down on the grill. Cook the vegetables turning them once or twice until grill marks appear, for about 4-6 minutes. Cook the salmon for 8-10 minutes without turning. In a salad bowl, mix together the vegetables and fish. Garnish with the basil and lemon slices.

WEEK 2

MONDAY

Breakfast: Mediterranean Omelet

Prep Time: 6-8 minutes

Total Time: 9-10 minutes

Nutritional Facts: 1 serving (302 calories per serving, 17 grams fat, 22 grams carbs, 18 grams protein)

Ingredients:

1 tablespoon feta cheese, crumbled

1 tablespoon heavy ream

2 eggs

1 tablespoon olive oil

salt & black pepper to taste

3 tablespoons pitted olives, sliced

2 artichokes, chopped

3 tablespoons tomato, diced

Directions:

Add olive oil to a small pan. Crack the egg and add the salt and black pepper and heavy cream. Once the egg starts to set, sprinkle with the olives, tomatoes, feta cheese and artichoke on half the egg. Fold the egg over. Cook the egg until completely set then remove from heat.

Lunch: *Mediterranean Chickpea Salad*

Prep Time: 12-14 minutes

Cook Time: 20-23 minutes

Nutritional Facts: 4 servings total (190 calories per serving, 8 grams fat, 29 grams carbs, 6 grams protein)

Ingredients:

2 cans chickpeas, rinsed and drained

.5 cup feta cheese, crumbled

.5 cup parsley, chopped

1 cucumber, chopped

8-10 cherry tomatoes, halved

13-15 pitted olives, sliced

1 bell pepper, chopped

.5 red onion, chopped

Dressing:

2 tablespoons extra virgin olive oil

a pinch of salt & pepper

2-3 cloves garlic, minced

.25 cup lemon juice

Directions:

In a large bowl, mix together the vegetables and chickpeas. Garnish with fresh parsley. Make your salad dressing in a separate bowl. Dress with the salad dressing and add feta cheese.

Dinner: One Pan Veggies & Baked Cod

Prep Time: 12-14 minutes

Total Time: 28-30 minutes

Nutritional Facts: 4 servings total (347 calories per serving, 23 grams protein, 19 grams carbs, 12 grams fat)

Ingredients:

2 cups cherry tomatoes

2 cups baking potatoes, diced

4 tablespoons olive oil

oregano & basil dried herbs to taste

salt & black pepper

1 pound cod fish divided into 4 pieces

Directions:

Pre-heat your oven to 400 degrees F. Add your diced potatoes on the baking tray. Season with olive oil, salt, black pepper, and herbs. Roast for 12-16 minutes in the oven. Remove from heat. Add tomatoes and fish pieces to the tray and drizzle with the leftover olive oil and any remaining spices. Bake the tray for another 10-12 minutes until the fish is cooked through.

TUESDAY

Breakfast: Fig Smoothie

Prep Time: 2 minutes

Total Time: 4-5 minutes

Nutritional Facts: 1 serving total (332 calories per serving, 79 grams carbs, 3 grams fat, 6 grams protein)

Ingredients:

6 fresh figs

.75 cup almond milk

.25 cup strawberries or berries of choice

1 banana

a handful of ice

Directions:

Blend everything smooth in a blender.

Lunch: Avocado, Smoked Salmon, and Cucumber Bites

Prep Time: 14-17 minutes

Total Time: 22-24 minutes

Nutritional Facts: 4 servings total (3 bites per serving, 212 calories per serving, 10 grams fat, 3 grams fiber, 6 grams carbs, 28 grams protein)

Ingredients:

a dash of black pepper

.5 tablespoon lime or lemon juice

1 avocado, peeled

1 large cucumber

6 ounces smoked salmon

chives or green onions for garnishing

Directions:

Wash your cucumber and slice into 12 .25" thick pieces and lay flat on a serving platter. Mash the avocado in a small and stir in the lemon juice. Create the snack by spreading some avocado on each cucumber then topping it with a thin slice of the salmon. Sprinkle some black pepper over each slice and top with the chives or green onion for garnishing.

Dinner: Mediterranean Stuffed Bell Peppers

Prep Time: 16-18 minutes

Total Time: 1 hour

Nutritional Facts: 6 servings total (280 calories per serving, 5 grams fat, 45 grams carbs, 15 grams protein)

Ingredients:

1 cup short grain rice, soaked in water

2.5 cups water

6 bell peppers, tops removed, cored

.5 cup chicken broth

1 cup chickpeas

.5 cup fresh parsley, chopped

.5 pound ground beef

.5 sweet onion, chopped

.5 teaspoon chili powder

1 tablespoon olive oil

.5 teaspoon paprika powder

salt & black pepper to taste

.25 cup tomato sauce

.5 teaspoon garlic powder

Directions:

In a medium pot, first add the olive oil and sauté the onions until golden brown. Cook the ground beef in the same pot. Season with salt, garlic, and black pepper, and add chickpeas. Add the rice, paprika, tomato sauce, and parsley to the pot. Then add water and chicken broth and let it simmer. Simmer and let everything cook for another 15 minutes until the rice is fully cooked. While the rice is cooking, grill the bell peppers for 10-12 minutes covered. Be sure to turn the peppers over so each side gets a consistent char. Remove from heat and let them cool.

Pre-heat your oven to 350 degrees F. Assemble the peppers in a baking dish by spooning the rice mixture to the very top of each pepper. Bake for 25 minutes with the tray covered in foil. Garnish with fresh parsley once removed from heat.

WEDNESDAY

Breakfast: Greek Tofu Scramble

Prep Time: 7-8 minutes

Total Time: 12-14 minutes

Nutritional Facts: 2 servings total (223 calories per serving, 14 grams fat, 11.8 grams carbs, 3 grams fiber, 12.8 grams protein)

Ingredients:

2 tablespoons lemon juice

8 ounces tofu

salt and pepper to taste

2 tablespoons olive oil

.5 onion, diced

2 tablespoons nutritional yeast

.5 cup bell pepper, diced

.25 cup fresh spinach, diced

3-4 cloves garlic, minced

.5 cup cherry tomatoes, halved

.25 cup pitted olives, sliced

Directions:

In a small bowl, crumble the tofu into bite-size pieces and mix with the lemon juice, and yeast, salt, and pepper. Add olive oil to a pan. Stir the garlic until its fragrant in the oil. Then add the onions, tofu, bell pepper and olives, stirring until well done. Add the basil and spinach. Stir until the spinach has reduced to half the amount. Lastly, add the cherry tomatoes and season your dish. Remove from heat.

Lunch: Peanut Butter & Banana Greek Yogurt Bowl

Prep Time: 3-4 minutes

Total Time: 8-10 minutes

Nutritional Facts: 4 servings total (363 calories per serving, 10.2 grams fat, 48 grams carbs, 36 grams sugar, 23 grams protein)

Ingredients:

2 medium bananas, sliced

.25 cup flax seed meal

1 teaspoon nutmeg or cinnamon powder

.25 cup natural creamy peanut butter or nut butter of your choice

4 cups vanilla Greek yogurt

Directions:

Divide the yogurt into four mason jars. Add the banana slices. Put your nut butter in the microwave for 10 or 15 seconds until it softens. Drizzle one tablespoon into each jar. Next, sprinkle some flax seed meal into each jar and top with a dash of cinnamon or nutmeg. You can keep these refrigerated overnight and have for breakfast throughout the week.

Dinner: Mahi Mahi & Vegetables

Prep Time: 8-9 minutes

Total Time: 25-35 minutes

Nutritional Facts: 4 servings total (308 calories per serving, 12 grams fat, 16 grams carbs, 36 grams protein)

Ingredients:

3 tablespoons olive oil, divided

.25 cup lemon juice

.25 cup fresh chives, minced

.25 cup pine nuts or nuts of choice

1 large onion, chopped

.5 pound Portobello mushrooms, chopped

salt and black pepper to taste

.75 cup bell pepper, chopped

4 6-ounce mahi mahi fillets (you can substitute with salmon)

Directions:

In a large skillet on medium heat, lightly fry the fish for 5-7 minutes in olive oil until the fish begins to flake. Remove from heat. Into the remaining oil, add the bell peppers, onions, lemon juice, and mushrooms. Season your vegetables. Add the fish on top and season the fillets with salt and black pepper. Cook for a little while longer until the fish is cooked through. Garnish with pine nuts and chives before serving. You can even toast your pine nuts for additional flavor.

THURSDAY

Breakfast: Mediterranean Breakfast Burrito

Prep Time: 12-14 minutes

Total Time: 28-32 minutes

Nutritional Facts: 2 servings total (1 burrito per serving, 248 calories per serving, 11 grams fat, 20 grams carbs, 14 grams protein)

Ingredients:

2 whole wheat tortillas

3 eggs

2 tablespoons sun-dried tomatoes, chopped

.25 cup canned beans

.25 cup feta cheese, crumbled

1 tablespoon pitted black olives, sliced

.5 cup fresh baby spinach, roughly diced

2 tablespoons olive oil

salt & black pepper to taste

Directions:

In a small saucepan on medium heat, add the olive oil and cook the eggs on both sides. Add the tomatoes, spinach olives, tomatoes and continue to stir. Season with pepper, salt and stir in the feta cheese. Heat up each tortilla in the microwave and divide the beans into each one. Divide the egg mixture into each tortilla. Grill on a panini press or lightly fry in a pan until golden brown.

Lunch: Almond & Orange Granola

Prep Time: 7-8 minutes

Total Time: 23-28 minutes

Nutritional Facts: 8 servings (.5 cup per serving, 239 grams per serving, 12 grams fat, 29 grams carbs, 6 grams protein)

Ingredients:

1 teaspoon ground cinnamon

.75 cup raw almonds

3 tablespoons olive oil

.5 cup honey or agave nectar

.5 cup golden raisins

.5 teaspoon sea salt

2 cups rolled oats

1 teaspoon orange zest

Directions:

First, pre-heat your oven to 350 degrees F. Combine oats, orange zest, almonds, and sea salt in a large bowl. Stir until all ingredients are combined. Pour in the honey and olive oil. Pour the granola out on the baking sheet and make an even layer. Bake for about 18-23 minutes. Halfway through, give the baking sheet a toss so everything will be evenly cooked. Remove from heat. Allow the granola to cool before adding in the raisins and breaking the granola into chunks.

Dinner: Olive & Lemon Chicken w/ Orzo

Prep Time: 12-14 minutes

Total Time: 25-30 minutes

Nutritional Facts: 4 servings total (324 calories per serving, 17 grams fat, 23 grams carbs, 27 grams protein)

Ingredients:

1 teaspoon dried oregano

.5 lemon cut into wedges

1 tablespoon lemon or lime juice

.75 cup uncooked whole wheat orzo pasta

1 can (~14 ounce) chicken broth

4 boneless chicken thighs (~1 pound total)

3 tablespoons olive oil

.5 cup pitted olives, sliced

Directions:

Add the olive oil to a large pan to lightly fry the chicken. Remove from heat. Add the chicken broth to the skillet and increase the heat. Cook until boiling and stir in the remaining ingredients until the liquid reduces. Add back in the chicken to the pan and cook until the pasta is tender.

FRIDAY

Breakfast: Ricotta Cheese & Fig Toast

Prep Time: 2-4 minutes

Total Time: 7-10 minutes

Nutritional Facts: 1 serving total (247 calories per serving, 30 grams carbs, 12 grams protein, 9 grams fat)

Ingredients:

pinch of sea salt

1 teaspoon almonds, sliced

1 fresh fig, or 2 dried ones sliced

.25 cup skim ricotta cheese

1 slice whole grain bread about .5" thick

Directions:

Toast your bread and top with the ricotta cheese, almonds, and figs. Add the sea salt for a pinch of contrasting taste.

Lunch: Brown Rice & Arugula Salad

Prep Time: 8-11 minutes

Total Time: 25-28 minutes

Nutritional Facts: 4 servings total (468 calories per serving, 21 grams fat, 48 grams carbs, 13 grams protein)

Ingredients:

1 package (~8 ounces) prepared brown rice

6 cups arugula

1 can (~15 ounces) garbanzo beans

.5 cup fresh basil, torn or roughly chopped

.5 cup cranberries

1 cup feta cheese, crumbled

Dressing:

.25 cup olive oil

a pinch of salt

3 tablespoons lemon juice

Directions:

Cook your rice according to its instructions and keep in a separate bowl. In another bowl, mix the cranberries, basil, cheese, garbanzo beans and arugula. In another small bowl, prepare your dressing and add salt to your taste. Add to your salad. Eat with the brown rice.

Dinner: Citrus Scallops

Prep Time: 18-20 minutes
Total Time: 36-38 minutes

Nutritional Facts: 4 servings total (238 calories per serving, 8 grams fat, 22 grams carbs, 21 grams protein)

Ingredients:
1 sweet pepper, sliced
1 pound sea scallops
5 green onions, chopped
salt & black pepper to taste
3 tablespoons olive oil
.25 teaspoon red pepper flakes
4 medium oranges, peeled and sectioned
2 teaspoons fresh cilantro or parsley, diced
3 tablespoons lime juice
2-4 cloves garlic, minced

Directions:
In a large skillet, lightly fry the onions, garlic, and pepper in olive oil until the vegetables are soft. Add the scallops and sprinkle with pepper, black pepper, and salt. Cook until scallops are cooked through. Add the lime juice. Reduce the heat before adding the orange slices and fresh cilantro. Cook until the scallops are lightly golden. Remove from heat.

SATURDAY

Breakfast: Whole Grain Oats & Raspberries

Prep Time: 11-12 minutes

Total Time: 13-15 minutes

Nutritional Facts: 1 serving total (283 calories per serving, 50 grams carbs, 12 grams protein, 8 grams fat)

Ingredients:

.5 cup whole grain oats

.75 cup raspberries (or berries of your choice)

.75 cup low-fat milk

Directions:

In a bowl, adds the oats and milk and top with the fruit.

Lunch: *Mediterranean Sweet Potato Hash*

Prep Time: 12-14 minutes

Total Time: 38-40 minutes

Nutritional Facts: 2 servings total (655 calories per serving, 25 grams fat, 99 grams carbs, 19 grams protein)

Ingredients:

1 cup shredded Mozzarella cheese

.25 cup pitted olives, sliced

salt & black pepper to taste

3 tablespoons olive oil

.5 teaspoon chili powder

3 cloves garlic, minced

1 onion, chopped

2 lemon wedges

1 cup pomegranate seeds

3 cups fresh spinach, chopped

4.5 cups sweet potatoes, peeled & diced

Directions:

In a large pan on medium heat, fry the potatoes in olive oil until cooked through. They should be light brown in color. This could take anywhere from 10-15 minutes depending on the thickness of your pieces. Once done, move to the back of the pan and add in the other vegetables. Once sautéed, add the minced garlic and season with salt, black pepper, and chili powder. Serve with Mozzarella cheese, pomegranate seeds, and lemon wedges.

Dinner: Cumin Beef Rice

Prep Time: 11-14 minutes

Total Time: 23-28 minutes

Nutritional Facts: 4 servings total (512 calories per serving, 17 grams fat, 53 grams carbs, 32 grams protein)

Ingredients:

1 green onion, chopped

2 cloves garlic, minced

.5 pound ground beef (or lamb)

1 tablespoon cumin

2 eggs

1 inch garlic piece, minced

3-4 cups rice, preferably a day old so it is less sticky

salt to taste

3 tablespoons olive oil

Directions:

In a large frying pan on medium heat, add the olive oil. Once hot, add the cumin and allow it to toast. You will see it turn brown and smell fragrant. Add in the ground beef and break up the meat. Stir and cook until it is cooked through. Add the salt, ginger and garlic and cook for another few minutes before adding the eggs. Swirl the yolk around so it mixes with the beef. Add the rice. Break up the bigger rice pieces until it is spread out evenly with the meat and egg. Remove from heat and garnish with green onion.

SUNDAY

Breakfast: Avocado Toast

Prep Time: 4-6 minutes

Total Time: 11-13 minutes

Nutritional Facts: 2 servings total (168 calories per serving, 10 grams fat, 16 grams carbs, 4.5 grams protein)

Ingredients:

2 cloves garlic, chopped

1 avocado, pitted, peeled, halved

1 tablespoon olive oil

4 pieces whole grain bread

salt & black pepper to taste

Directions:

Mash your avocado so it's chunky. Season with salt and black pepper. Toast your bread pieces and rub each side with the garlic until fragrant. Brush with the olive oil. Divide the avocado to two pieces of toast to form two sandwiches.

Lunch: Sweet Potato Wedges w/ Tahini Sauce

Prep Time: 12-14 minutes

Total Time: 28-30 minutes

Nutritional Facts: 2 servings total (290 calories per serving, 44 grams carbs, 6 grams protein, 8 grams fiber, 11 grams fat)

Ingredients:

2 sweet potatoes

salt & black pepper to taste

.5 teaspoon paprika powder

2 tablespoons tahini sauce

.5 teaspoon chili powder

.5 teaspoon cumin

1 tablespoon olive oil

Directions:

First, pre-heat your oven to 400 degrees F. Wash and scrub the sweet potatoes and cut into 4-6 wedge pieces. Arrange on the baking tray and drizzle with the olive oil, paprika, chili powder, salt, and black pepper. Roast in the oven for about 30-40 minutes until they are crispy on the outside and still tender in the inside when you use a fork to cut open. Remove from heat. Let cool and serve with tahini sauce.

Dinner: Chopped Chickpea Greek Salad

Prep Time: 7-9 minutes

Total Time: 15-18 minutes

Nutritional Facts: 2 servings total (521 calories per serving, 62 grams carbs, 16 grams protein, 20 grams fat)

Ingredients:

.5 avocado, pitted and diced

.5 cup black olives, sliced

.5 red onion, sliced

.5 cucumber, sliced

.5 can chickpeas

3 cups fresh baby spinach, roughly chopped

.5 bell pepper, sliced

1 cup cherry tomatoes, halved

Dressing:

4 tablespoons olive oil

a pinch of sea salt

.25 teaspoon Italian seasoning

.5 teaspoon mustard

2 teaspoons lemon juice

1.5 tablespoon balsamic vinegar

Directions:

Mix together the salad dressing ingredients. Add the spinach to a salad bowl. Layer all your prepared veggies and chickpeas on top. Add the avocado and dressing and toss well to combine.

What are some healthy snack recommendations on the Mediterranean diet? Here are some suggestions!

- Pita bread and hummus: Hummus is a versatile dip you can use on burgers, salads, or as a dip with whole grain chips or pita bread. It's great to dip vegetables in too! You can switch up your hummus flavors but using different things like spicy jalapeno, red pepper, or sun-dried tomatoes.

- Olives

- Fresh greens smoothie

- Dates or figs: These are true Mediterranean fruits and can help satisfy your sweet tooth!

- Whole grain crackers with goat cheese: Be sure you're consuming whole grain crackers which will be healthier than refined bread ones.

- Fresh fruit: An easy and sweet option, this is better for you with natural sugars instead of refined sugars you can find in baked goods.

- Nuts and seeds: These are a great source of unsaturated fat and can boost your cardiovascular health. When having nuts, be sure you're eating the raw version instead of an unhealthy candied or salty version with unnecessary calories.

- Fruit slices with almond butter: As we stated that nuts are healthy, nut butter is a great option too! Be sure there are no additional preservatives or sugar in your butter. Try and buy organic so you're getting the best ingredients.

- Greek yogurt with fruit or nuts: Greek yogurt is a great source of probiotics. Be sure you're using the plain version with no flavoring. Add your own fresh fruit or nuts to add flavor.

- Fruit with ricotta cheese spread: This is another healthy alternative to cheese that you can eat with various fruits.

- Crackers with tangy cheese and salty olives: Combining sweet and salty tastes is a great way to satisfy your taste buds and reduce any cravings.

- Sun-dried tomatoes with goat cheese

- Whole wheat crackers with tuna

- Whole grain granola: You can make your own homemade granola so you are aware and in control of what ingredients you are using. Try finding wholesome ingredients like raw nuts, chia seeds, and flaxseed.

- Roasted chickpeas: Find healthy recipes where you can roast chickpeas with spices, paprika, or cinnamon.

- Hard-boiled eggs: Be sure you aren't going over your egg intake for the week!

Conclusion

Thanks for making it through to the end of *Mediterranean Diet*. We hope this book was informative and was able to provide you with answers and a thorough introduction to the Mediterranean diet. When starting a new diet and lifestyle change, it's important to conduct research and learn about the background, health benefits, and a guide to what you can and cannot eat. The Mediterranean diet is all about making a healthy lifestyle change that you can maintain long-term. It's not meant to be a "quick fix" diet to drop some pounds. If you truly capitalize on the diet and follow it religiously in your life, you can experience the many astounding health benefits that have been researched which includes lowering your cholesterol, preventing the onset of Type 2 diabetes, losing weight the right way, and protecting your cells from unnecessary stress.

As we said, the Mediterranean diet is not just a dietary adjustment, but a complete lifestyle change. Ancel Keys was the first to notice the link between the people of the Mediterranean's heart healthy diet and longer lifespan. In order to correctly emulate that, we must improve not only our diet, but our physical activity as well. The people of the Mediterranean incorporated exercise into their routine regularly, and it's important that we try and do the same. It doesn't have to be a set workout time at the gym, but rather taking a walk around the neighborhood or taking a long bike ride can help you burn calories and spur weight loss. Weight loss can only occur if you are following a calorie deficit diet. Even if the Mediterranean diet is easy to follow in the sense that it doesn't require counting carbs or calories, it's still important you're aware of your portion size, snacking, and caloric intake if you want lose weight. That can only happen if you're burning off more calories than what you're taking in!

So many diets fail because people focus on what they cannot eat. With the Mediterranean diet, there is a wider variety of food that you are allowed to eat! Though you should try and limit your dairy, red meat, and poultry intake, there are still many delicious meals you can prepare. You can still eat a red meat or a chicken dish once a week, but try and use leaner cuts of meat and be conscious of your portion size. Incorporate more fish into your diet and have fresh fruits and vegetables on hand to create a quick salad. Also, remember that you should use extra virgin olive oil in your cooking and in your salad dressing. It's heart healthy and packed with antioxidants that keep your cells healthy and prevent inflammation in the body.

With a 14-day meal plan included, we have recipes to help you plan your meals for breakfast, lunch, and dinner! With a shopping list of Mediterranean diet ingredients to bring home, you can whip up these recipes using fresh vegetables, herbs, whole grains, and fish that you've bought. If you make the effort to incorporate exercise into your routine, you'll truly be gaining the long-term health benefits that this diet promises.

Finally, if you found this book useful in any way, a review is always appreciated!

Author email:

eathealtyeat@gmail.com

Visit the author's facebook page:

https://www.facebook.com/EatingHealtyEating

Mediterranean Diet Cookbook

Healthy and tasty recipes to get you started

Table of Contents

Mediterranean Diet Cookbook   (Book n.2)

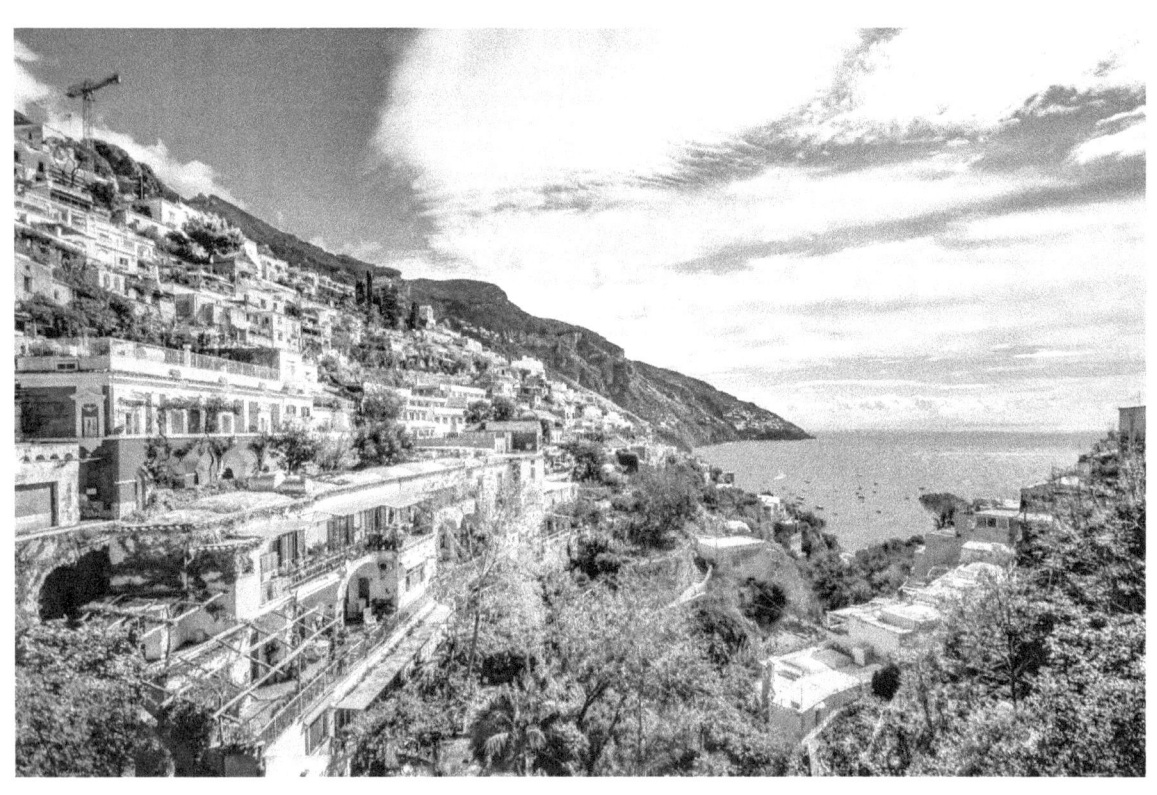

(Amalfi Coast – Italy)

Introduction & Disclaimer

Congratulations and thank you for downloading *Mediterranean Diet Cookbook*: *healthy and tasty recipes to get you started.*

First things first... let's get started with an overview of what the Mediterranean diet actually *is*, where it comes from, and how it can help you live a better life! Over the past few decades, the Mediterranean diet has become increasingly known - and popular - in the United States and in the rest of the world... and this for a good reason.

The Mediterranean diet is not just a weight loss regime; it is indeed a complete lifestyle, based on virtuous eating habits, physical activity and top-quality foods, that can improve your overall health. This diet is based on fruits and vegetables, healthy fats and lean meats, and if you get your basics right, you won't need to worry about sticking to a strict diet or counting your calories: you will be able to eat delicious and inspiring dishes every day, improving your health and your well-being. It is a healthy, balanced lifestyle that you can easily follow; the key is just to remember what you should and should not eat, and how often, and to combine this way of eating with an active lifestyle and general good habits.

This book aims to provide a simple overview of the Mediterranean diet, its characteristics and the health benefits it can bring you. It also includes a section on which items cannot miss in your kitchen and a set of inspiring tasty and healthy recipes to help you plan and prep your meals and ease into the Mediterranean diet lifestyle.

Please keep in mind that this lifestyle change, like any other diet you choose to follow, should not be started without consulting your personal doctor or GP. Your GP can examine your overall health and medical needs to make sure that there are no contraindications and that this lifestyle change will not harm you. All information provided in this book is purely illustrative, only aims to provide information, and does not constitute medical advice.

There are plenty of books on this subject on the market, so thanks for choosing this specific one!

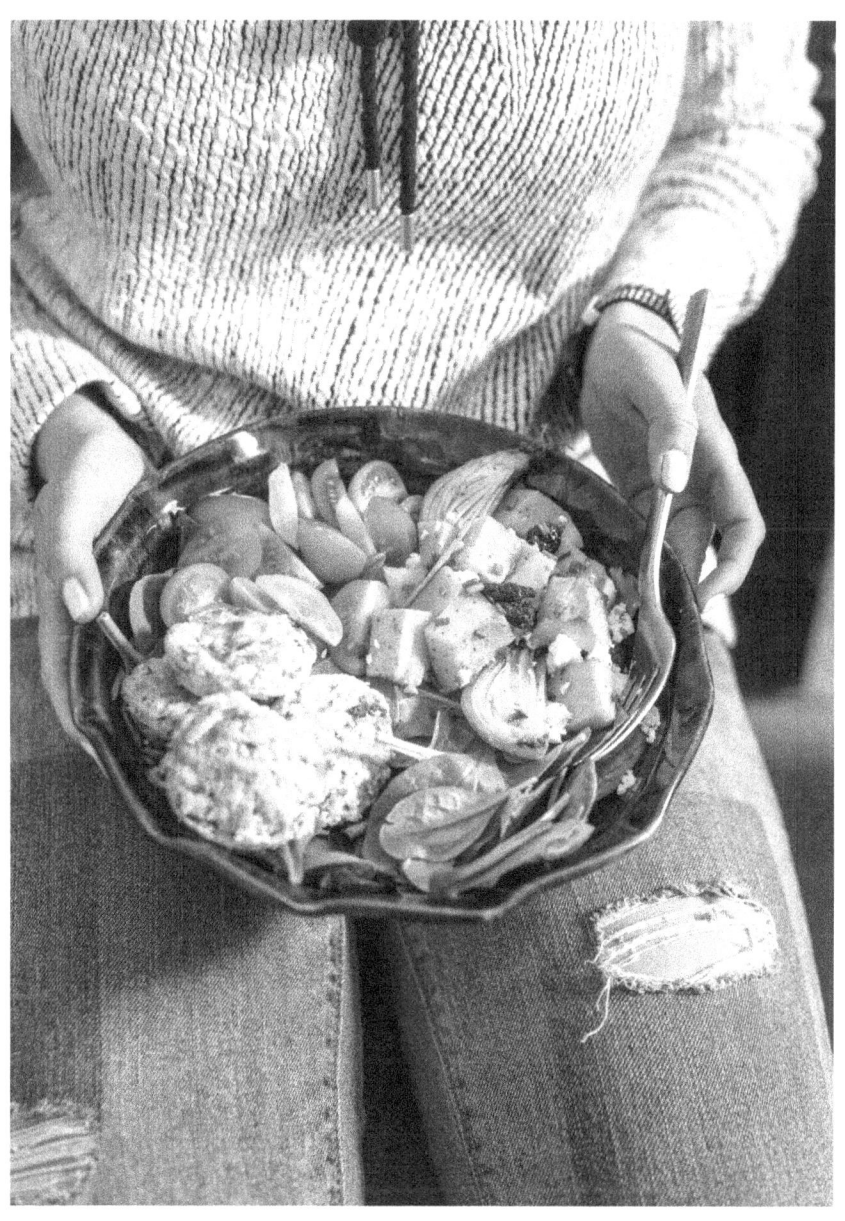

More than a simple diet - a lifelong way of eating, of considering food that comes with a whole lifestyle of its own.

Picture a village by the sea, its narrow streets lined with white or pastel-colored houses leading straight up to the water. Picture endless stretches of olive trees and maritime pines along winding dirt roads. Picture a family cooking dinner in a small kitchen with green shutters: someone is kneading dough for pasta or bread, someone else is chopping tomatoes for the sauce, another person stirs a pot, they chat or sing.

Cooking and eating is a joyful affair; eating well brings happiness, in addition to improving your health, especially so if you share this passion and these moments with the people you care about.

Based on these beliefs, the Mediterranean diet is not a weight-loss plan per se; it is a type of eating pattern that arises from the history and lifestyle of the countries around the Mediterranean Sea, and more specifically Italy, Southern France, Greece and Spain. It is based on fresh produce, whole grains, legumes as well as the healthy fats that are contained in olive oil or certain types of fish. Being that it is not a fixed regime but a lifestyle that automatically leaves out certain unhealthy foods, this diet will open up possibilities for millions of recipes that will improve your health without ever making you feel like you are "on a diet" as we usually intend it. In the Mediterranean diet, quality should always be preferred over quantity; whenever possible, it is recommended to only choose seasonal fresh produce (straight from the farmer's market), organic products, local meat. Your meals should try to revolve around seasonal ingredients - choosing seasonal produce is the more sustainable choice, as it cuts down on transportation or cultivation costs, and it will save you some money too!

When Shopping for products that can't be locally sourced, it is crucial to read the nutritional labels carefully, to make sure that you are not buying something filled with preservatives or refined sugars.

Indeed, the Mediterranean diet is, and has long been, one of the healthiest diets on the planet, with impressive results on the overall physical and mental health of those who follow it.

This lifelong habit can't be reduced to picking a number of recipes or sticking to a certain amount of calories; the Mediterranean lifestyle typically includes regular exercise in the daily routine (be it just a brisk walk or bicycle ride to work, or going for a hike or swim on the weekends when the weather allows for it), as well as healthy and consistent sleeping patterns. Consistently eating the right meals at the right time is also fundamental; typically, you will also choose smaller portion sizes than we might be used to. This, however, doesn't mean that you will be starving yourself: if you eat foods that are "filling" or rich in fiber, you will feel full and satisfied even though you are consuming a much smaller amount of calories or fats.

Mediterranean meals tend to be long, quiet moments of relaxation with family or loved ones, which perhaps include cooking together or just sitting down for a long chat while you eat. While this can be difficult or impossible to fit into a busy day-to-day life, with fixed working hours and a million things to take care of, it's always good to remember to take your time! There's nothing like a quick-fix snack or a hurried meal on your feet to worsen your health and your eating habits.

Always try to find even just a few moments to sit down and enjoy your meals. A great part of the Mediterranean diet and lifestyle relies on this - tasting and savoring the food, and the moments.

One more thing to keep in mind is that there is no one, specific way to follow the Mediterranean diet and lifestyle; there are no fixed plans that are 100% guaranteed to make you lose weight. On the other hand, there are basically no foods you won't be allowed to eat at all (while there are some food types that should be eaten rarely or in moderation), and the freedom provided by this type of eating habit will make it possible for nearly everyone to find a diet that best suits their health, their needs and their goals.

As for can't-miss foods, the Mediterranean way of eating revolves mainly around healthy foods, chock-full with vitamins and nutrients, such as fresh vegetables (leafy greens, onions, carrots, eggplants...) and fruits (apples, grapes, oranges...), legumes (beans, lentils, chickpeas), whole grains, fresh fish, EVO (extra virgin olive) oil, nuts and seeds (almonds, walnuts, sunflower seeds...). Seafood and fish should be eaten at least twice weekly.

Dairy products (especially cheese), goat milk, eggs, and white meat should be consumed in moderation, while red meat only rarely (once a week tops, for example). Foods that are too rich in sugar or that are processed or refined should be avoided as much as possible, such as sugary snacks or candy, refined grains, packaged meat etc.

It is also quite easy to swap out these unhealthy foods for healthier versions: choose whole-wheat or whole-grain bread and pasta over white ones, extra virgin olive oil over soybean oil or margarine, natural brown sugar over refined white sugar.

For instance, you should always choose EVO oil when cooking, rather than refined oils or other fats such as butter or margarine; EVO (extra virgin olive) oil is an unprocessed olive oil, extracted with natural methods and not refined or diluted with other oils. It is very nutritious, as it contains vitamins E and K as well as plenty of high-quality compounds called phenols, that have antioxidant qualities. Antioxidant means that they protect molecules from the chemical process called oxidation, that causes damage to the cells in our body. By eating the right foods, cooked in the right way, we can have access to a whole range of nutrients that improve our body's health.

As mentioned before, this is not strictly speaking a weight-loss diet - the kind of eating regime you force yourself to follow for a while before going back to your previous habits, which is bad for your health as much as for your self-esteem! The Mediterranean diet is a style of eating that, once you have made it yours, will allow you to eat a variety of delicious and satisfying foods that never leave you feeling "starved" or deprived. This way, you are also less likely to fall back on random or unhealthy snacking between meals. If you wish to make the most of the health benefits of this diet, more about which you will find in chapter 2 below, and use it to keep your weight in check as well, here are a few things to keep in mind.

First of all, keep an eye on your portion sizes; focus on the Quality rather than on the quantity. By choosing a smaller portion and eating more slowly, you will feel full sooner, and still feel satisfied! Also, certain foods are more "filling" than others, and can leave you feeling full and content, and less likely to reach for a snack soon after. For example, vegetables such as kale or broccoli are rich in fiber and have less calories compared to meat or other food types.

It is also important to avoid skipping meals whenever you possibly can: science tells us that if we eat too long after the previous meal, or when we are particularly hungry, we will take in an excess amount of calories. This also goes for shopping... if you go grocery shopping when you are feeling hungry, the risk of reaching out for foods that look inspiring and tasty at the moment is so much higher, but you'll regret it later! For this reason, it is important to plan meals or even prep them in advance, so that you can organize your shopping as well, and to set aside the time for each meal or snack.

You might want to get into the habit of setting aside an hour or so at night to prep your food for the next day; this will allow you to always have a healthy and nutritionally satisfying meal at hand, without having to fall back on quicker snacks or unbalanced foods. You may also just prepare larger portions of whatever you are having for dinner and save the leftovers for lunch.

While it is always better to eat fresh and tasty meals, remember that many foods can also be frozen and stored in the freezer; their preservation times vary depending on the ingredients, so you will need to be careful and not let things sit around for too long, but this is a great way to store foods that take a long time to prepare! There are a few rule of thumbs that you can follow: first of all, never place cooked food in the fridge while it is still hot! Let the leftovers cool then divide them into individual portions and freeze them. The portions must be placed inside airtight containers or tightly wrapped in freezer bags. Make sure to always defrost your food completely, either by moving it to the fridge for as long as it takes, or in the microwave; heat well before eating. You should avoid cooling and reheating food more than once, and once you defrost the leftovers you should heat and eat them within 24 hours.

If you tend to eat out a lot, please don't feel like you should stop doing it or avoid certain types of foods or restaurants: eating out in good company is a wonderful way to spend time and enjoy meals! Once you get into the spirit of the Mediterranean diet, you will notice just how simple it is to follow even when you are not making your own food at home. Probably any restaurant menu has a variety of offerings from which you will surely be able to pick something that is good for your eating habits. In general, try to avoid fast foods or large, cheap restaurant chains that tend to use pre-cooked or frozen foods and lower quality ingredients. Aside from that, just keep an eye out for your Mediterranean diet staples: any dish based on a variety of veggies, pasta dishes, fish courses will likely be easy to find and not drift too far from your preferred diet! Also remember that the Mediterranean diet welcomes having a glass or two of wine with your meals (unless you should avoid it for various medical or social reasons). Don't be afraid to enjoy a good dinner with your friends!

One more thing - to embark on your Mediterranean diet journey, you should be willing to make certain changes such as clean up your kitchen or pantry removing the refined or processed foods you may have stored aside over time. Below in chapter 4 you will find examples of shopping lists or the staples that can't miss in your home.

You should also try to incorporate vegetables, fruits or whole grains in all your meals and snacks, as these fiber-rich foods will, as mentioned above, help you feel full longer. The same goes for protein-rich food such as beans, eggs, fish and nuts. If you often feel like having a snack between meals, don't stock up your pantry with sugary snacks, candy bars or extra-savory potato chips: you won't need or miss them at all! Walnuts, almonds, sunflower seeds, pumpkin seeds all make for tasty and filling snacks, as does dried fruit (raisins, dates) or fresh fruit; if just biting into a whole apple doesn't sound appealing to you, there are a million alternatives that you can try - pre-chopped carrot and celery sticks, mixed berries to eat with Greek yoghurt... You can also make your own chip-substitute by baking slices of other vegetables such as carrots, kale leaves or even apples with a bit of olive oil and salt!

In general, eating and planning your diet should not be something that stresses you out; it should be a natural and pleasant part of life, that can be shared with the ones you love. Shopping together at a local market, picking out each ingredient individually, choosing a recipe and cooking together all make for lovely moments of bonding or relaxation as well.

Love your food, love yourself: eating well can make you happy!

Chapter 2: Health Benefits of the Mediterranean Diet

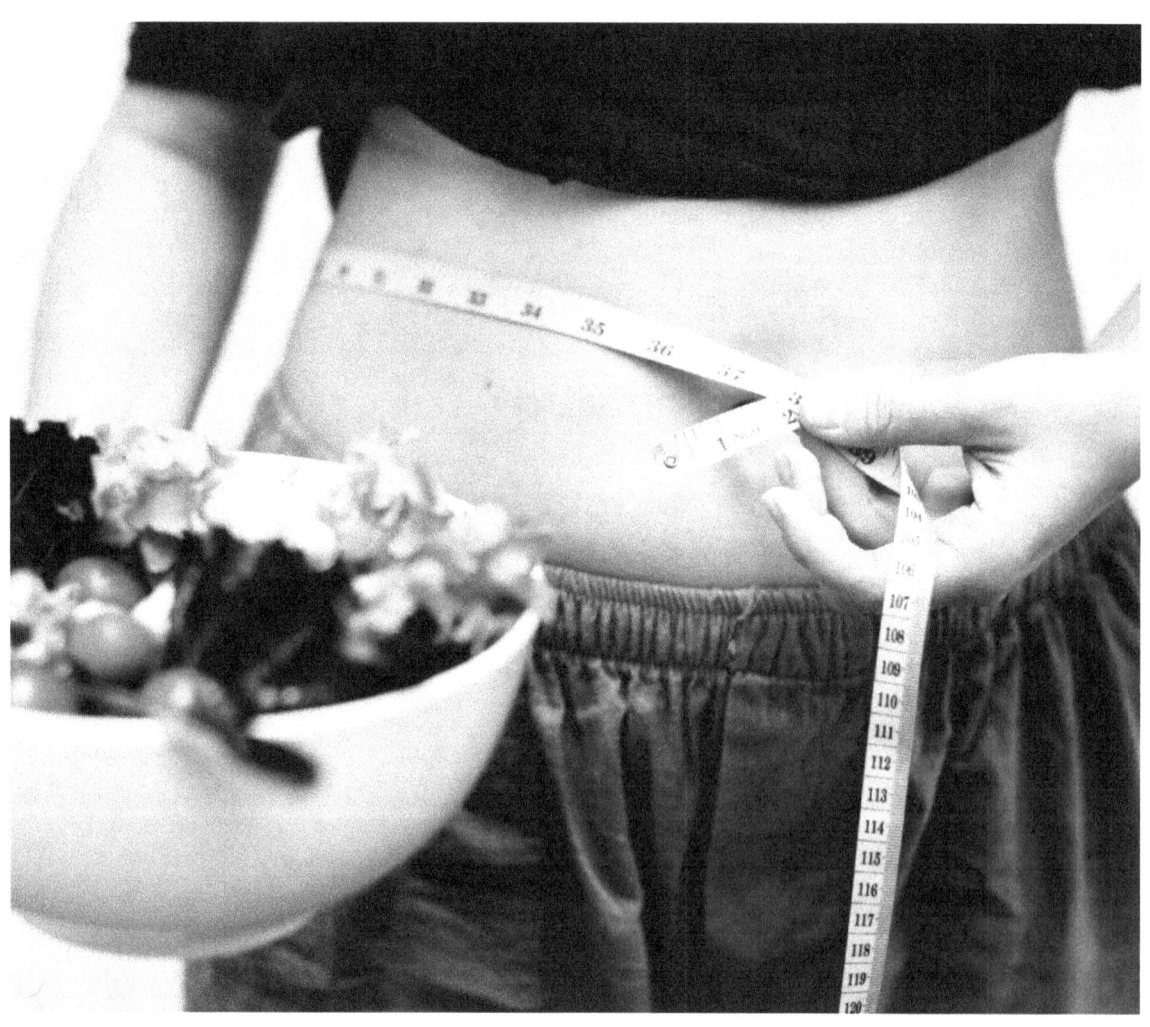

The Mediterranean diet and eating regime is good for your whole body, from your brain to your bones.

That's right: not only it can help you lose weight, but it can improve your mental and physical wellbeing, reducing the risk for cardiovascular disease, depression, type 2 diabetes and so much more!

There has been a lot of research and study into the traditional Mediterranean diet, taking off from the fact that several scientists noticed that people in Mediterranean countries tended to be healthier and to have longer life spans compared to residents of other parts of the world, notably the United States. In the 1950s, American scientist Ancel Keys compared the health of citizens living in poorer areas of Italy to those of the wealthiest New Yorkers and found that the first were in exceptionally better health. Thus Ancel Keys studied these populations and their eating habits, as well as their overall lifestyle. He found out that the people in the Mediterranean regions were consuming healthy fats such as those contained in olive oil, nuts, fresh fish, thus resulting in better heart health and, in general, longer lives.

The Mediterranean diet as we mean it today, that began to become popular in the United States in the 1990s, is focused on the traditional foods that those people used to eat and the lifestyle that they used to live. The "good" foods are paired with regular physical exercise and, in general, a healthy lifestyle and habits.

Further research into this way of eating has shown that it can produce weight loss results, as well reduce the risk of developing conditions such as type 2 diabetes, high cholesterol and high blood pressure.

The healthy fats contained in EVO oil or nuts, compared to more processed fats, help reduce cholesterol levels and Decrease the risk for cardiovascular disease. Indeed, out of all types of diets, the Mediterranean regime is the most helpful in reducing high triglyceride levels (that can lead to high cholesterol and an increased risk of heart disease), while maintaining "good" cholesterol (HDL cholesterol) that comes from beneficial monounsaturated and polyunsaturated fats. These healthy fats can improve cellular function in the body as well as overall heart health.

Furthermore, the Mediterranean diet has a higher proportion of unsaturated fats compared to saturated fats and tends to avoid over-processed foods; for this reason, this diet also improves Blood sugar levels. Maintaining lower insulin levels and blood sugar levels can delay or hold back the onset of **type 2 diabetes**. It can also fight diabetes by enabling you to lose weight in a healthy way, that doesn't depend on counting your calories or starving yourself, but on paying better attention to what you eat and how much of it. You will avoid processed or refined foods and always pick fresh vegetables over red meat or snacks... This is especially true when you pair the healthy eating regime with an active lifestyle that can burn off excess weight. Also, the foods typically recommended in the Mediterranean diet are rich in fiber, which slows digestion and prevents spikes in blood sugar levels.

The Mediterranean diet also protects Cognitive health: the healthy fats in the Mediterranean diet, as well as the anti-inflammatory properties of fresh produce, have an incredibly beneficial effect on the brain's nerve cells - they prevent them from deteriorating with age. This means that the Mediterranean diet could help prevent the onset of neurodegenerative conditions such as dementia or Alzheimer's.

Similarly, the antioxidants contained in fruits and vegetables, as well as the omega 3 fatty acids contained in fish, can have a beneficial effect in **improving your vision**. Studies show that 1 serving of fish a week could be enough to lower the risk of developing eye damage. Nuts and seeds also contain fatty acids that protect the cells in the eyes from being damaged by age.

Cutting out refined sugars and replacing them with natural sugars, like those found in fruit, also helps Maintain skin health and prevent common skin conditions like acne or eczema. The antioxidants in fresh fruit and vegetables keep a healthy glow on your skin and can actually make you look younger!

In general, the benefits of antioxidants and substances that reduce inflammation in the body can Keep our cells healthy, somewhat preventing the damages that come with aging and helping us keep active for longer.

The combination of these factors can actually mean that the Mediterranean diet, if followed consistently and paired with regular physical exercise and good life habits, will not only help you lose weight; it can actually **increase your lifespan** and help you live a longer, healthier life.

No one diet is the right solution for everyone, and of course there may not be a 100% correspondence between following the Mediterranean diet and seeing all these health improvements; in case of doubt, please do not hesitate to consult with your GP or to look into the more specific studies on this research! However, it can be said for sure that the Mediterranean eating regime, compared to most other diets, has the greatest benefits on your health.

Chapter 3: The Main Meals

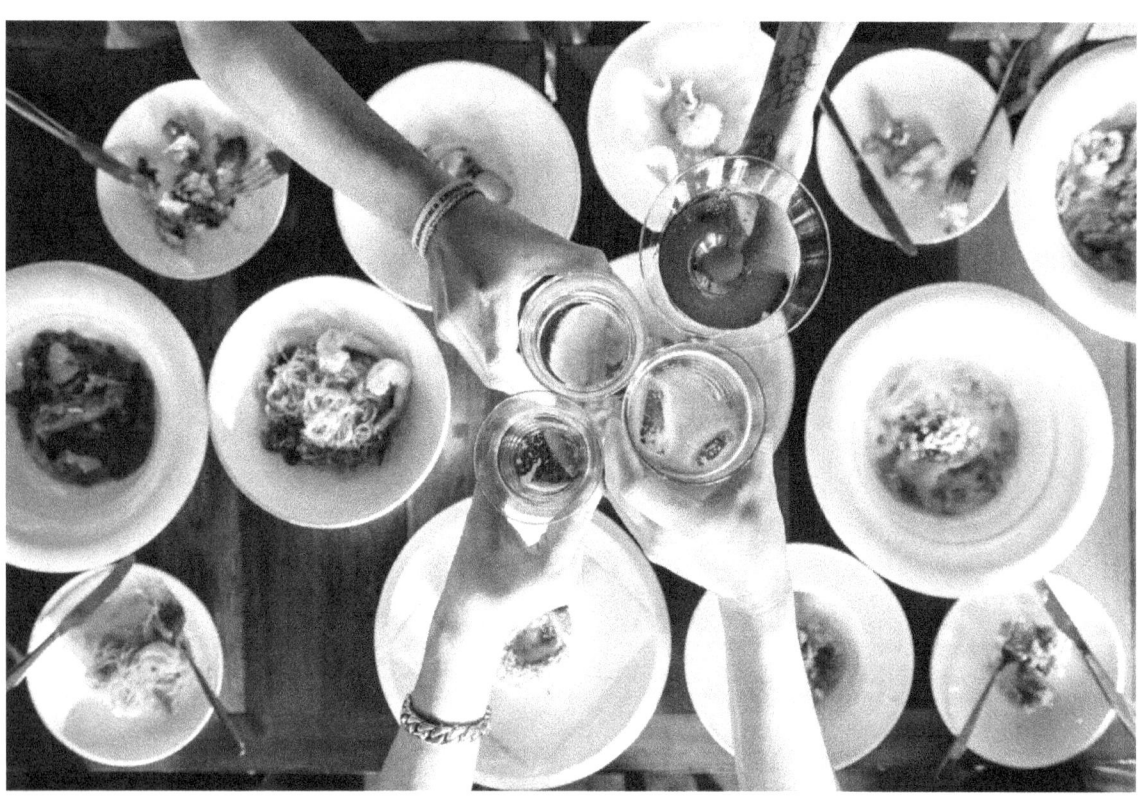

The Mediterranean diet is focused around three main meals, and small (optional) healthy snacks in between. The three meals are, perhaps obviously, breakfast, lunch and dinner.

It is important to not skip any meals and to try to keep your eating schedule regular, with meals 4-5 hours apart and smaller snacks in between so that you never feel starved or aching for food. If you eat when you are too hungry or your body is deprived of certain nutrients, you will be more likely to reach for the "wrong" type of food, like snacks rich in sugar that give you an instant rush by causing a spike in your blood sugar levels, but leave you feeling hungry and tired again soon after.

The key to making this eating regime work, and to gain all the benefits it can have on your health and on your weight loss as well, is to be consistent, to plan ahead, to work prepping/planning meals into your daily routine as naturally as possible. It shouldn't feel like too much of an effort or a waste of time; try to find the joy in choosing a recipe, picking the ingredients, finding the magic of cooking so that you are creating something delicious - and good for you!

Breakfast is an extremely important meal. First of all, fitting the time for breakfast into your daily routine can help enforce a positive lifestyle; it can even motivate you to get up a bit earlier to make time for this meal - and who knows, a quick pre-breakfast workout or walk outside... Forget about just rolling off the bed and straight to work while grabbing a cup of coffee on the go! In fact, breakfast should give you all the energy you need to face the day after a good night's rest, but it should also be a time you take to think about the day that lies ahead, or talk with a loved one or family member. It's a healthy, positive moment in your daily routine. Be it five minutes before rushing off to work or a long lazy Sunday brunch, it is always the meal that sets the mood for the rest of the day!

A balanced breakfast should give you a decent caloric intake, amounting to 15-20% of your daily quota; it should be tasteful, filling and rich in vitamins, fibers and carbs. A breakfast too rich in sugars or fats will leave you feeling hungry again too soon after, and may result in unhealthy snacking before lunch. A simple but balanced breakfast, however, will help you feel full and energetic until lunch and set a positive trend for the next meals as well.

Typically, the Mediterranean breakfast includes foods from each of these three groups: dairy (milk, yogurt, kefir), fruit (fresh seasonal fruit, jam, fresh-pressed orange juice), cereal (whole-grain bread, cereal, muesli). There are many ways to combine these ingredients in quick and simple or more elaborate ways. Remember that your fruit can come in any shape: fresh, in a fruit salad, pressed in juice, dried... Just make sure it's not too full of extra sugar.

Lunch should make up a pleasant and satisfying break in your day. Forget about grabbing a sandwich on the go; whenever possible, try to find a slot in your day to dedicate to just eating your lunch. If you are at work, you should drop everything else, look away from the computer, take those 15 minutes or half an hour to eat your food and relax for a moment. Lunch is often considered the most important meal of the day; it is not uncommon for workers in the Mediterranean region to close shop for two-three whole hours and go home to share a meal with the rest of the family! Of course this is not always feasible, but still, it's good to enjoy lunch - and with the recipe suggestions below, you surely will!

Your lunch should be filling, but not so much that it leaves your stomach stuffed and your mind clouded for the rest of the afternoon. Salads, whole-wheat pasta or rice, and plenty of fiber-rich vegetables are all great ingredients. You can also incorporate healthy proteins into your lunch, such as legumes or white meat.

Dinner can be similar to lunch as for recipes and nutrient intake. You should try to avoid foods that are harder to digest, which could result in a bad night's sleep, and try to eat at least two hours before your usual bedtime. Avoid caffeine at night, while a glass or two of red wine can easily fit into your meal, unless it is not advisable due to specific medical or lifestyle reasons. Mediterranean dinners often include hearty soups, pasta dishes, bakes.

Snacks can be consumed in moderation, mid-morning or mid-afternoon. Avoid store-bought sugar-filled snacks and candy whenever possible, give your preference to nuts and seeds or fresh fruit that can give you the "good" sugar and fats you need to keep going without giving you sugar rushes. Great snacks that you can prepare in advance and always have ready at hand are mixed nuts (almonds, walnuts, cashews), sliced carrots or fennel, fresh apples or bananas, mixed berries, etc.

Throughout the day, remember to drink plenty of fresh water; coffee or tea are also accepted, in moderation, while packed fruit juices or sugary drinks such as sodas should be avoided.

Chapter 4: Shopping List and Kitchen Staples

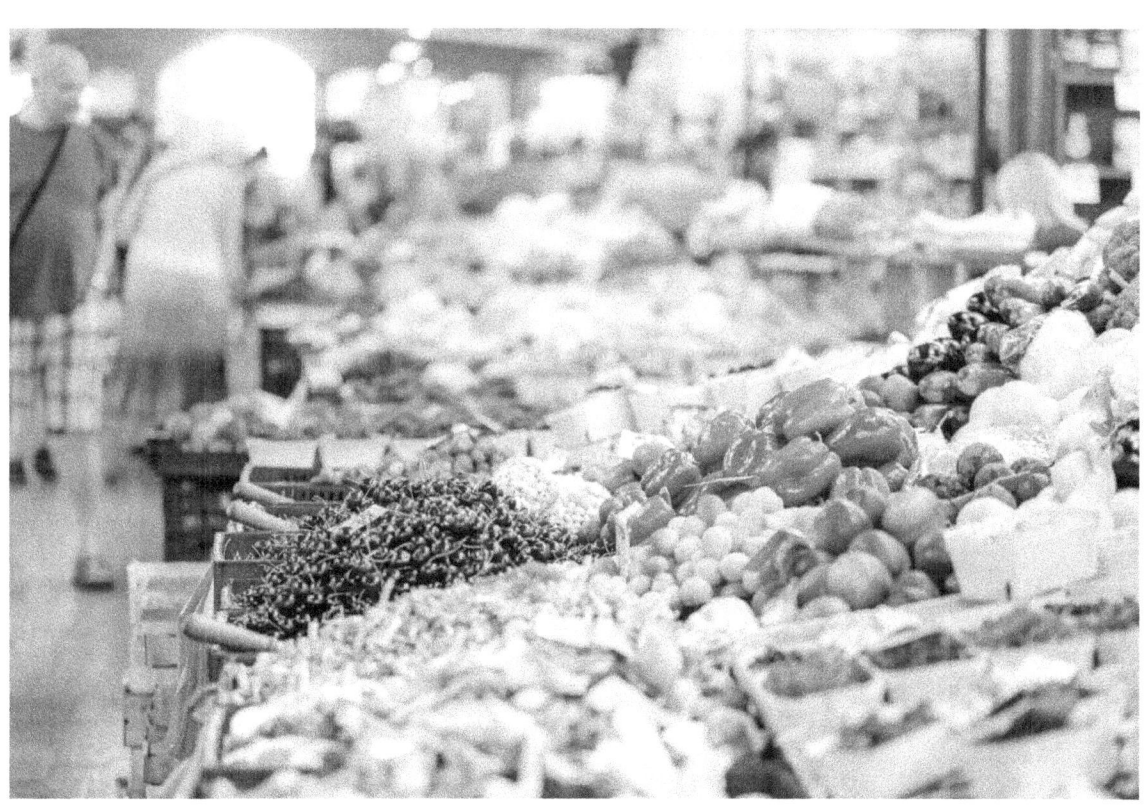

As mentioned in the first chapter, the Mediterranean diet is based on a specific pyramid of foods that should be eaten daily, often, with moderation or rarely.

The base of the pyramid, meaning those foods that can be consumed daily and abundantly, is made up of foods from plant sources such as **olive oil, fruits, vegetables, whole grains, legumes, nuts and seeds, spices and herbs.** The guidelines for healthy dieting, regardless of the geographical area, suggest having between 6 and 12 servings of fruit and vegetables per day; this means that each meal you cook or eat should include a few variations of these items. The only fat you use in cooking should be olive oil, rather than butter or margarine; spices and herbs (either fresh or dried) are great for adding flavor to your food without having to use too much salt. Fresh herbs are also quite easy to grow on your windowsill if you feel up to a little gardening and want a supply of fresh basil and sage always at hand!

Below is a list of items your kitchen should never be without.

- *Extra virgin olive oil* is one of the staples in your pantry. It is the healthiest, least processed version of olive oil and contains high levels of antioxidants. Use it to cook, fry, season or just drizzle over your dishes.
- *Vegetables*: from tomatoes and bell peppers to zucchini, eggplant, cauliflower, spinach, there is an endless variety of vegetables to choose from! When possible, prefer seasonal vegetables or ones sold from local farmers, so you will be sure that they have not been treated with preservatives - and you will save money as well. Combine veggies however you please, raw or cooked, in salads, smoothies, soups, stir-fries, by themselves or as sides.
- *Fruits*: a great alternative to sugary snacks or desserts, they can be a real treat in themselves. A wide variety of fruits gives you a wide range of vitamins, minerals and other nutrients. If you are looking to lose weight, give your preference to fruits that are low in sugar such as oranges, grapefruits, apples or pears.

- *Legumes*: beans are an excellent source of high-quality protein as well as folate, calcium, iron and zinc. Also, they are rich in fiber, which means that eating them can give you strength and help you feel full for longer. You can use them in soups, to make dishes such as hummus, or paired with veggies or other ingredients.
- *Nuts and seeds*: walnuts, cashews, almonds, sunflower seeds, chia seeds: these "superfoods" are all rich in fiber and nutrients. Any mix of these is perfect as a healthy snack in between meals or incorporated into other types of dishes. Chia seeds are especially packed with nutrients (fiber, protein, fat, calcium, manganese...) and loaded with antioxidants, in a tiny amount of calories. They are almost flavorless and can be easily fit into many types of recipes, both sweet and savory.
- *Whole-grain flour, bread, cereal*: forget white refined grains and open up to a whole world of whole grains: whole-wheat pasta or bread, barley, quinoa, non-processed cereal... All super healthy and satisfying to eat. A smaller portion leaves you feeling full for longer, compared to their refined alternatives.
- *Herbs and spices* should never be lacking in your pantry! They are perfect for adding flavor to any dish you make, without using too much salt or sugar; also, most herbs and spices contain healthy compounds that may help reduce inflammation and the consequent damage to cells, such as phytochemicals. Dried herbs work just as well! Any Mediterranean cook always has ready at hand a variety of spices and herbs, from cardamom to cloves, cumin to turmeric, bay leaves, coriander, garlic powder, oregano, rosemary, thyme...

A key element in the Mediterranean diet is to keep yourself hydrated by drinking lots of **fresh water** during the day. Carry a bottle with you at all times and refill it whenever you get the chance! In fact, water is essential, among other things, to ensure that your kidneys and other bodily functions work just fine; it is also necessary to help carry oxygen throughout the body, to boost skin health, and to properly dissolve and make accessible the minerals and nutrients contained in the food we eat. If you get "bored" with regular water, you can try adding some flavor to it by infusing lemon slices, cucumber or even strawberries. Try to stay away from sugary sodas or packed fruit juices that are often rich in sugar and calories.

The Mediterranean diet also recommends a moderate consumption of **wine** with meals. Moderate being the key word, which means 1 glass a day for women, 1-2 glasses for men. If there are individual health or family reasons for which you should not drink any wine or alcohol, avoid it and please refer to your doctor in case of doubt.

***

According to the Mediterranean food pyramid, **fish and seafood** should be consumed two or three times a week as a great protein source. Mediterranean fish are also rich in omega 3 fatty acids, that are extremely beneficial for your health. Buy the fresh fish you find at the market, or frozen fish, or even canned fish such as sardines or anchovies; don't be afraid to experiment and choose new types of fish and seafood such as shrimp or crab.

Dairy products, eggs and poultry should be consumed with moderation, not on a daily basis. If you wish to eat them more often, choose low-fat dairy products and "healthier" products such as Parmesan, feta, Greek yogurt. Eggs can be eaten alone or used in baking or cooking. If you wish to eat poultry several times during the week, turkey is a healthier, leaner alternative to chicken.

Red meat should be consumed very rarely, and even then, in small quantities and choosing lean cuts with little fat. After all, you are already getting your daily protein intake from other plant-based sources! Avoid processed or packaged meat like hot dogs or sausages.

You should also try to avoid **sugars** (candy, chocolate, sodas), that you can substitute with fresh fruit or berries, and all types of **highly processed foods**; this is why you should always read the labels carefully before buying your food.

Remember to always check for the quality of the products you are buying and, when you have the chance, try to shop at local markets or to buy locally-sourced foods.

Stock up your pantry with a nice basis of Mediterranean staples: EVO oil, canned beans/chickpeas/lentils, canned tuna or preserved fish, oil-preserved vegetables, whole-grain pasta, nuts and seeds, spices and herbs. If you do so, it will then be much easier to plan your shopping as you will only have to buy the fresh ingredients you need for your day-to-day meal prep!

Also, it is a good idea to plan your meals at least a few days ahead, so that you can get all the ingredients you'll need at once, and have time to prep some things in advance.

The rest of the book is made up of a series of recipes and cooking inspirations, many of which can be prepared in advance and eaten over several days too.

Don't be afraid to experiment, to try out the endless possible combinations of ingredients and flavors, to mix styles and cooking methods and you will never get bored with your Mediterranean diet.

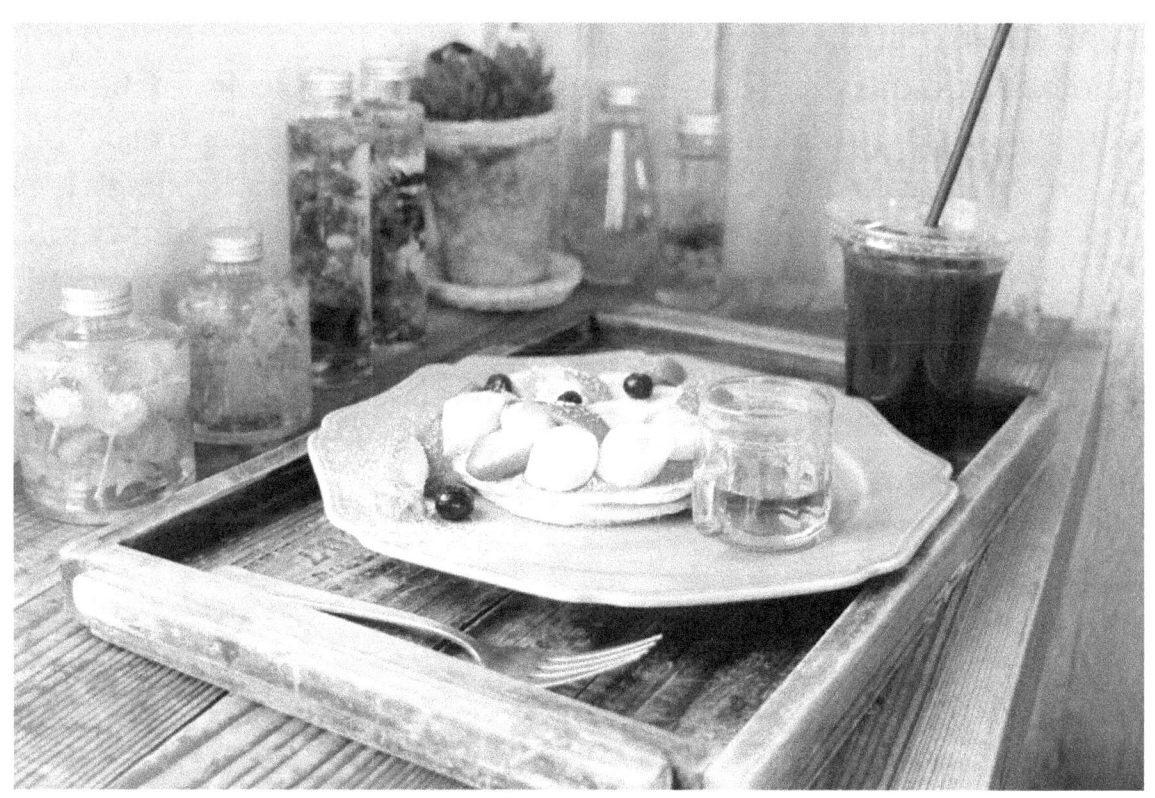

MEDITERRANEAN BREAKFAST BOARD

Let's start off this section on the most important meal of the day with something that is not so much a recipe, as an idea for a tasty and healthy breakfast that you can assemble however you please.

Imagine a table set up with a nice wooden board on which you place bowls and plates of delicious and nutritious items: a combination of soft cheeses and Greek yoghurt that you can serve with a drizzle of honey or olive oil for a more savory taste, toasted whole-grain bread or flatbread, a little bowl of hummus, and all the seasonal fruit you like, sliced or diced, or dried fruit as well. If you are aiming to lose weight, give your preference to fruits that contain less sugar, carbs and calories such as berries, grapefruits, oranges, etc.

As mentioned before, the Mediterranean breakfast typically includes foods from three main groups: dairy, fruit and cereal. The dairy can consist of milk, yogurt, Greek yogurt, kefir or soft cheeses such as labneh or ricotta; fruit can come in any shape and size (fresh, sliced, pressed, dried...); as for cereal, you can choose toasted whole-grain bread, flatbread, quinoa, muesli or oatmeal... Anything you like!

Listed below are three examples, arranged by prep time, that you can choose from if you just have a few minutes before you run off to work or it's a lazy Sunday and you can take your time, perhaps surprise your friends or family with a lovely breakfast board...

BREAKFAST BOARD IDEA #1
Prep time: 5 minutes
4 slices whole-grain bread, fresh or toasted
1 cup Greek yoghurt
Dried fruit, a handful of one or more types (walnuts, almonds, dates, figs...)
Muesli cereal/rolled oats with milk

BREAKFAST BOARD IDEA #2
Prep time: 10 minutes
4 slices whole grain bread, toasted

1 cup soft cheese (eg. labneh, ricotta, halloumi)
Seasonal fresh fruit, sliced or diced
Honey

BREAKFAST BOARD IDEA #3
Prep time: 20 minutes
4pcs flatbread (see recipe below)
1 cup hummus (see recipe below)
1 cup soft cheese (eg. labneh, ricotta, halloumi)
Honey
Seasonal fresh fruit, sliced or diced
Dried fruit, a handful of one or more types (walnuts, almonds, dates, figs...)
Fresh-pressed orange juice

Flatbread
Ingredients:
1 cup whole-wheat flour
1 cup Greek yoghurt
⅓ tsp bicarbonate

You can very simply make your own flatbread with just three ingredients and a few minutes' prep time!

Mix the whole-wheat flour, the Greek yoghurt and the bicarbonate in a bowl; mix and knead for 2-3 minutes until the dough is nice and smooth. Split the dough into 4 equal-sized parts and flatten each part with a rolling pin. Heat up a non-stick pan on high heat and cook the flatbreads for 1-2 minutes on each side. Once they are done, you may brush them with a mix of melted butter and herbs.

Hummus
Ingredients:
1 can chickpeas, drained and rinsed
½ tsp baking soda
2 lemons, pressed
1 clove garlic, minced
½ cup tahini (sesame seed paste)
2 tbsps cold water
1 tbsp EVO oil
Salt, cumin, paprika to taste
Fresh parsley, chopped

All you need to do is add the ingredients to the food processor in the right order! First, whip the tahini and lemon juice for 1 minute; then add the olive oil, minced garlic, salt and blend for 30 seconds; add the chickpeas next (in two parts for a smoother result) and blend for a few more minutes. Add 2 or 3 tablespoons of water to reach the right consistency. Adjust with salt if needed; serve with a dash of paprika and cumin, a drizzle of EVO oil and a sprinkle of chopped parsley.
Hummus can be stored in an airtight container in the fridge for up to 1 week.

FETA QUINOA MUFFINS

Ingredients for 12 muffins:
1 onion, finely chopped
1 cup cherry tomatoes, chopped or sliced
1 tbsp fresh oregano
2 tsps EVO oil
6 eggs
1 cup cooked quinoa
1 cup feta cheese
Salt and pepper

Prep time: 15 minutes - Cook time: 30 minutes

Nutritional values per serving: Calories 429 - Fat 24g - Carbs 33g - Protein 20g

Preheat the oven to 180°C/375F. Sauté the onions in EVO oil in a skillet for a few minutes, then add the tomatoes and let fry for another minute or so. Remove the skillet from the heat and stir in the oregano, salt and pepper to taste. Pour the eggs in a mixing bowl and blend them with the quinoa and the crumbled feta cheese. Then add the tomatoes and onions and stir. Pour the mixture into a paper-lined (or silicone) muffin tin and bake in the oven for 30 minutes or until a toothpick comes out clean. These muffins are delicious both warm and cold, and are great to prepare in advance and have ready at hand the next day. Extra tip: You may also replace the tomatoes or combine them with other veggies to your liking: baby spinach, fresh mushrooms or kale all work great!

BAKED EGGS AND AVOCADO TOAST

Ingredients for 2 servings:
2 eggs
1 avocado
2 slices whole wheat bread
1 tsp lemon juice
1 tsp soy sauce (optional)
Salt and pepper

Prep time: 10 minutes - Cook time: 5 minutes

Nutritional values per serving: Calories 337 - Fat 25g - Carbs 20.5g - Protein 11g

Avocado toast is quite popular right now, but in this recipe it's paired with eggs, for a stronger kick. A fun way to have eggs for breakfast!
Smash the avocado in a small bowl with the lemon juice and a pinch of salt. Fry the eggs in a nonstick pan with just enough EVO oil to coat the bottom; cook until the whites are set but the yolk is still runny. While the eggs cook, toast the bread in another pan. Then spread the avocado on the bread and place one egg on top of each slice. Season to taste with salt and pepper and a dash of soy sauce if you wish.

APPLE AND BANANA QUINOA BOWL

Ingredients for 4 servings:
1 cup quinoa
1 ½ cups water
2 apples, diced
1 banana, sliced
1 handful almonds, chopped
Honey

Prep time: 5 minutes - Cook time: 25 minutes

Nutritional values per serving: Calories 390 - Fat 15g - Carbs 57g - Protein 11g

Quinoa is a hypocaloric and gluten-free ingredient, rich in fiber and protein, ideal to start your day!

To make this breakfast bowl, first of all, peel and core the apples and dice them.

Place the quinoa, the water and the diced apples in a saucepan and bring to a boil. When the water boils, cover the pan and lower the heat; let it simmer for approx. 25 minutes. After this time the quinoa will have absorbed most of the water.

Transfer into a large bowl (or two smaller ones) and let it cool slightly.

Peel and slice the banana and add it to the quinoa and apple mixture. Chop up the almonds and add those as well. Drizzle with honey and serve!

You may also add other fruits to the bowl, such as fresh strawberries or dried coconut. Get creative: this base works well with a variety of different options!

OVERNIGHT OATS

Ingredients:
Rolled oats or muesli
Nuts (walnuts, almonds)
Chia seeds
Milk (almond, coconut or cow)
Fresh fruit (berries work best!)
Honey

Prep time: 5/10 minutes - Total time: 12 hours

Nutritional values per serving (approximate; may vary depending on chosen ingredients): Calories 209 - Fat 8g - Carbs 27g - Protein 7g

A healthy breakfast idea that doesn't require any cooking and can be assembled quickly the night before. They can be stored in the fridge for up to five days, so you could also make a batch on Sunday night and have breakfast ready all week long!
Just layer the ingredients in a mason jar or airtight container: first the oats and the seeds/nuts, then pour the milk and drizzle the honey on it, and top with the berries. Sliced fruits such as bananas or apples are fine if you plan on just eating them the next day, but they won't store as well for more days. You can also use frozen fruits, especially raspberries/blackberries.

WHOLE-WHEAT BERRY MINI MUFFINS

Ingredients for 12 muffins:
2 cups whole-wheat flour
1 cup brown sugar
1 tsp salt
1 tsp baking soda
1 cup blueberries or strawberries
½ cup EVO oil
1 cup plain yogurt

Prep time: 5/10 minutes - Total time: 12 hours

Nutritional values per serving (2 muffins): Calories 430 - Fat 17g - Carbs 61g - Protein 7g

Delicious muffins that will entice kids and adults alike, for a sweet breakfast or snack.

Preheat the oven to 180°C/375F.

In a large mixing bowl, combine all the dry ingredients, sifting the flour to avoid any clumps. Add the blueberries (whole) or the strawberries (chopped) to the dry mixture.

In another bowl, whisk the EVO oil with the yogurt. Pour the liquid ingredients over the dry ingredients and stir to combine. When you have a smooth batter, prepare the muffin tin by greasing it or lining it with parchment paper or liners. Fill each place with batter, almost up to the top. Sprinkle with a dash of brown sugar and/or cinnamon if you wish.

Place in the oven and bake for approx. 20 minutes or until a toothpick comes out clean. Once they are cooked, transfer to a rack to cool. They last several days at room temperature, but you can also wrap them in wax paper or put them in an airtight container and freeze for longer storage.

PEANUT BUTTER AND BANANA TOAST

Ingredients for 4 servings:
4 slices whole-wheat bread
½ cup peanut butter
1 or 2 bananas, sliced

Prep time: 5 minutes - Cook time: 5 minutes

Nutritional values per serving: Calories 311 - Fat 17g - Carbs 31g - Protein 12g

This may sound and look like a sugary snack, but it's actually a smart breakfast choice! The whole-wheat bread gives you fiber and vitamins, keeping you full and active throughout the morning; peanut butter is rich in healthy fats and protein, while bananas contain large quantities of fiber and potassium.
This recipe couldn't be simpler: you just have to toast the bread to your liking, spread the peanut butter, and add the banana slices. You may sprinkle with cinnamon for extra flavor.

COCONUT DATE BITES

Ingredients:
½ cup cashews or walnuts
12 dates, pitted
½ cup dried coconut, shredded
1 tbsp water
1 tbsp EVO oil

Prep time: 10 minutes (plus cooling)

Nutritional values per serving: Calories 234 - Fat 15g - Carbs 25g - Protein 4g

Get all the energy you need with these bite-sized treats! A great addition to your breakfast, but you can also carry them around with you as snacks, for example after a workout or when you need an extra energy boost. Rich in vitamins, fiber and minerals (selenium, potassium, magnesium), dates are an excellent resource in your Mediterranean diet.

First off, place the nuts in your food processor (use cashews or walnuts depending on your taste) for approx. 15 seconds. Then add in the pitted dates, half your shredded coconut (so ¼ cup), 1 tablespoon of water and 1 of EVO oil. Process for a while, until you get a smooth but not too soft mixture. The mixture should have the right consistency for you to be able to roll it in your hands and make it into a ball.

As you make the bite-sized balls, roll them in the remaining shredded coconut and place them in a baking tin or on any flat surface that will fit in your fridge. The balls should rest in the fridge for at least an hour before eating them, as this will allow the ingredients to bond and hold together. After one hour, when they have hardened enough, you can transfer them to an airtight container or freezer bag to save space, and store for several days!

ITALIAN APPLE TART

Ingredients for 1 tart:
For the pastry:
2 cups flour
1 ½ sticks butter
1 tbsp sugar
1 egg yolk
½ cup cold water
Salt

For the frangipane base:
½ cup butter
½ cup sugar
2 tbsp flour
1 cup almond paste
1 egg + 1 egg yolk

For the filling:
4-5 red apples
Sugar as needed

Prep time: 30 minutes - Cook time: 40 minutes

Nutritional values per serving: Calories 622 - Fat 44g - Carbs 54g - Protein 5g

This apple tart, while not exactly calorie-free, is a delicious and healthy(ish) addition to your breakfast or afternoon snack.

Start by preparing the pastry: sift the flour and mix it together with the butter, the sugar and the egg, mixing until it resembles coarse sand. Add 2 tablespoons of milk and a pinch of salt and toss a while longer, until it forms a ball. Wrap in plastic wrap or wax paper and leave to rest for 30 minutes in the fridge. (You may also use a store-bought tart shell).

Preheat the oven to 200°C/400F.

While the dough is resting, prepare the frangipane base. To make frangipane, cream the butter and sugar in a mixing bowl, then add the rest of the ingredients and blend until smooth. You may also use a whisk to smooth the mixture out (or the whisk attachment in your food processor).

Butter a tart pan, roll the pastry dough and place it in the pan. Prick the pastry with a fork so it doesn't puff while baking. Cover the pastry base with the frangipane base.

Peel and slice the apples into thin half-moon shapes that you will then arrange over the base, slightly overlapping, in concentric circles. Sprinkle the apples with sugar. Fold over or trim any excess pastry.

Bake at 200°C/400F for 15 minutes, then lower the temperature to 180°C/375F and bake for another twenty minutes or until the apples are perfectly soft when pierced with a toothpick.

Remove from the oven and let the tart cool off in its pan.

SAVORY RICOTTA MUFFINS

Ingredients for 12 muffins:
2 cups fresh ricotta
4 eggs
8 cherry tomatoes
4 tbsps olives, chopped
Fresh basil leaves, chopped
Salt and pepper to taste

Prep time: 5 minutes - Cook time: 20 minutes

Nutritional values per serving: Calories 288 - Fat 15g - Carbs 16g - Protein 21g

A healthy and filling savory breakfast or snack that only takes a few minutes to prepare.

Preheat the oven to 180°C/375F. Whip the ricotta in a mixing bowl, beat the eggs into it, then add the chopped cherry tomatoes, olives and chopped basil leaves. Season with salt and black pepper.

Line a muffin tray with papers and fill each one equally. Bake for approx. 20 minutes, until the tops turn golden brown or a toothpick comes out clean.

As an extra tip, you can certainly wrap the muffins up individually in wax paper or muffin liners and bring them with you as a ready-to-go snack.

BERRY BANANA SMOOTHIE

Ingredients for 1 smoothie:
1 banana
2 cups berries (strawberries, raspberries, blueberries)
1 cup milk
½ cup oatmeal

Prep time: 5 minutes

Nutritional values per serving: Calories 474 - Fat 9g - Carbs 88g - Protein 16g

A super quick and simple breakfast idea, that combines fresh fruit, rich in antioxidants and vitamins, with oatmeal, for all the nutrients and fibers you need to start the day. A splash of color and flavor for your morning!
Just combine the ingredients in the blender and... mix!
This smoothie also lends itself to a million different interpretations: you can replace the berries with apple slices, pineapple chunks, sliced peaches... You may also use almond milk instead of regular milk for an even healthier alternative.
Extra tip: if you want your smoothie to be cold and thicker, freeze the fruit (sliced or chopped up) overnight.

SHAKSHUKA BREAKFAST EGGS

Ingredients for 4 servings:
4 large ripe tomatoes
4 eggs
1 onion, chopped
1 cup tomato sauce
1 tbsp tomato paste
Powdered cumin
Powdered chili pepper
Powdered sweet paprika
1 clove garlic
Fresh coriander
EVO oil

Prep time: 20 minutes - Cook time: 35 minutes

Nutritional values per serving: Calories 129 - Fat 5g - Carbs 16g - Protein 9g

This simple Middle-Eastern dish is an excellent way to incorporate eggs into your weekly meal plan. Eating eggs for breakfast gives you all the proteins you need for the day - plus it tastes delicious!
To make shakshuka, first grab your food processor and blend one peeled clove of garlic with 3 tablespoons chili pepper, 1 tablespoon sweet paprika powder, a dash of salt and 1 or 2 tablespoons of olive oil, until you get a paste. This typical paste from Libya is called **felfel u ciuma** and can be stored in an airtight container in the fridge for several months. Prepare a jar in advance and always have it ready at hand!

In a large skillet or frying pan, heat up 2 tablespoons EVO oil with one tablespoon of felfel u ciuma and one tablespoon of powdered cumin. Mix thoroughly for a few minutes, then add one tbsp tomato paste. Wash, peel and dice the tomatoes (to peel them more easily, you can dunk them in boiling water for a few seconds).

Chop the onion and add it into the skillet along with the diced tomatoes and one cup of tomato sauce. Cook on moderate heat for 10 minutes. Then break the eggs straight into the pan and cook according to your taste.

Serve with a garnish of fresh coriander leaves.

ZUCCHINI AND CARROT FRITTERS

Ingredients for 4 servings:
2 zucchini
2 carrots
1 green onion
½ cup chickpea flour
½ tsp baking soda
½ tsp baking powder
2 tbsps EVO oil (plus more for cooking)
2 tbsps Greek yogurt or ricotta cheese
Salt and pepper to taste

Prep time: 15 minutes - Cook time: 10 minutes

Nutritional values per serving: Calories 200 - Fat 9g - Carbs 23g - Protein 9g

A weight loss-friendly, healthy idea for breakfast that you can also prep in large batches in advance!
First off, whisk the yogurt or ricotta with EVO oil then add the chickpea flour, the baking soda and baking powder and mix until smooth.
Peel the carrots and shred the carrots and the zucchini, then pat them with a clean dish rag to remove excess water. Peel and chop the onion.
Toss the vegetables in the bowl with the other ingredients.
Heat a skillet on medium heat and coat the bottom with some olive oil (a few tablespoons should do). When the oil sizzles, drop a small scoop of mixture into the skillet and flatten it out. Let cook a few minutes then turn over to finish cooking.

If you want to store them for later, let the fritters cool and then freeze them in individual plastic bags or wrapped in foil.

Chapter 6: Lunch

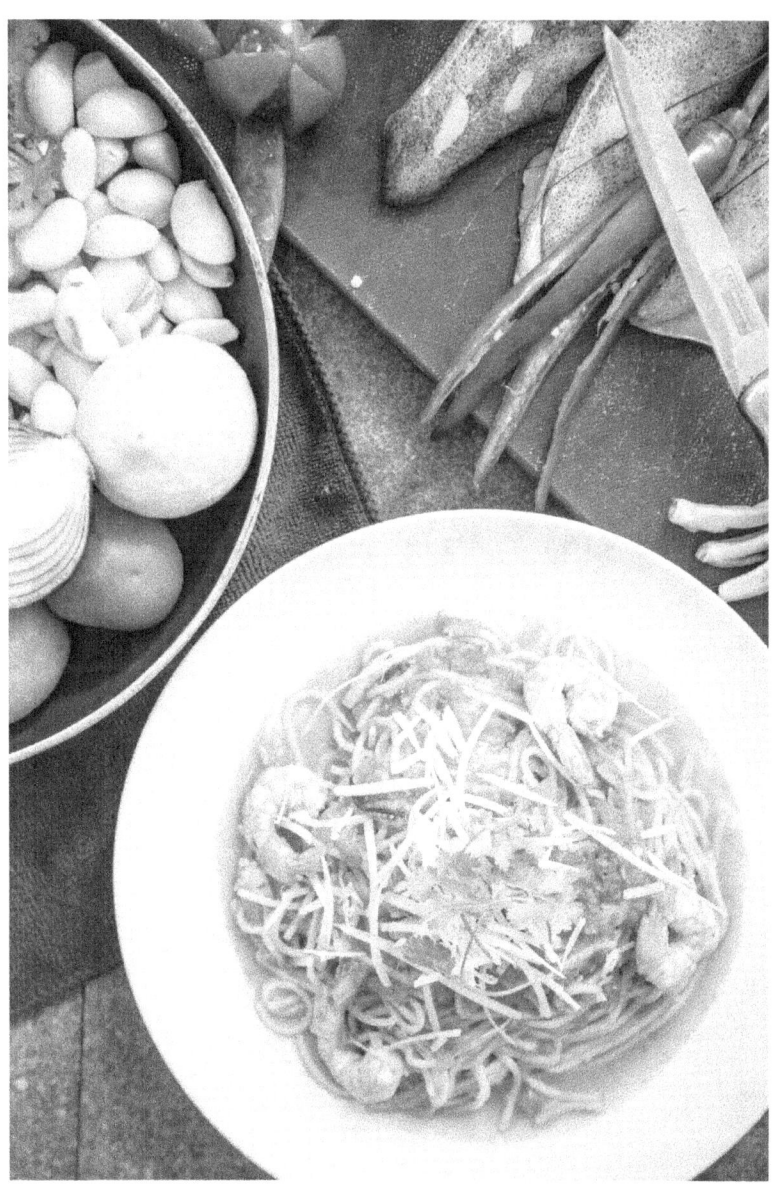

BRUSCHETTA WITH CHEESE AND TOMATOES

Ingredients for 4 servings:
4 slices whole-wheat bread
2 cloves fresh garlic
2 cups cherry tomatoes, chopped
A handful of fresh basil leaves
EVO oil
Salt and pepper
1 cup fresh ricotta

Total time: 20 minutes

Nutritional values per serving: Calories 173 - Fat 6g - Carbs 18g - Protein 12g

A light lunch that tastes like summer!
Toast the bread in a toaster or frying pan, without adding any fats, then rub the fresh garlic on it.
Dice up the tomatoes and season them with just a drizzle of EVO oil, some chopped basil leaves and a dash of salt; leave them to rest and soak up the flavor for a few minutes.
In the meanwhile, spread the fresh ricotta on the toasted bread, then arrange the tomatoes on top and serve.
Add basil leaves as garnish for an extra touch of color.
Bruschetta is best made on the spot and eaten fresh!

HORIATIKI SALAD

Ingredients for 4 servings:
4 large ripe tomatoes, chopped
1-2 cucumbers, sliced
1 small onion, diced
1 green pepper, chopped
1 cup feta cheese
2 dozen black olives
Chopped parsley or oregano
¼ cup olive oil
1 lemon, squeezed
2 tbsps vinegar
Salt, pepper

Total time: 20 minutes

Nutritional values per serving: Calories 305 - Fat 25g - Carbs 12g - Protein 8g

A typical Greek salad perfect for a hot summer day or whenever you crave that refreshing taste!
Cut the tomatoes in wedges and slice the cucumber. Cut up the pepper and the onion in rings. Mix all the ingredients in a large bowl.
In another bowl, make the lemon vinaigrette by whisking the oil with the vinegar and the lemon juice, then adding salt and pepper. Pour this dressing on the salad. Dice the feta cheese and add it to the salad, along with the olives. Add parsley or oregano, as you prefer, and serve cool.

One good thing about this salad is that it actually stores well in the refrigerator for several days; just remember to store it in an airtight container, and to store the vinaigrette in a separate jar.

PANZANELLA

Ingredients for 4 servings:
6/8 slices of stale bread
White wine vinegar
2 ripe tomatoes, chopped
15 leaves of basil
1 cucumber, chopped
1 large red onion
Salt, pepper
Ground thyme
Ground marjoram

Prep time: 15 minutes

Nutritional values per serving: Calories 192 - Fat 2g - Carbs 34g - Protein 10g

This dish unites all of Central and Southern Italy and was historically invented to use up stale bread, but it is still so tasty and healthy!

Peel the onion and slice it thin, then soak in a bowl with water and a tablespoon of white wine vinegar (the longer it soaks, the better).

Peel and slice the cucumber and set it aside. Then wash and chop the tomato, removing its seeds, and set it aside as well.

Now take the slices of stale white bread, remove the crust with a knife, then sprinkle them with a mixture of water and vinegar - they just need to be moist, not soaked. When the bread has softened, squeeze any excess water out of it and break it up roughly with your hands into a large salad bowl. Add the onion, the tomato, the cucumber and the chopped basil leaves to the bread.

Gently mix the ingredients with a wooden spoon, drizzle with olive oil, then season to taste with salt, thyme, marjoram. Let it rest in the fridge for at least one hour (but the longer the better) so that the bread soaks up all the taste.

Extra tip: prepare this recipe in a jar or lunch box at night, and have it ready to go for lunch the next day!

ORANGE FENNEL SALAD

Ingredients for 4 servings:
3 fennel bulbs
6 ripe oranges
Fresh mint leaves
1 tsp dried oregano
2 tbsps EVO oil
Salt and pepper

Prep time: 15 minutes

Nutritional values per serving: Calories 245 - Fat 7g - Carbs 45g - Protein 5g

This salad is full of vitamin and nutrients, and if you pair it with whole-grain crackers or breadsticks, it can make for a filling lunch as well!
Peel the oranges, removing the pith as well, then slice them and remove the seeds. Arrange the slices in a salad bowl and season with a dash of salt and freshly ground black pepper. Shave the fennel with a peeler and slice it. Mix the oil, vinegar, oregano and mint leaves in another bowl and soak the fennel in it. Add the seasoned fennel to the oranges. Tip: This salad tastes better if you leave it to rest for a few hours and let the oranges soak up the flavor. Just assemble the ingredients in the morning before you leave for work and enjoy it at lunch!

SEASONAL VEGGIE PASTA BOWL

Ingredients for 4 servings:
14-16 oz whole-grain pasta
Fresh seasonal vegetables
2 carrots, chopped
2 pieces of celery, chopped
1 white onion, chopped
EVO oil
A few anchovy fillets (optional)
Salt, chili pepper

Prep time: 5-10 minutes - Cook time: 15 minutes

Nutritional values per serving (approximate, may vary depending on chosen ingredients): Calories 307 - Fat 9g - Carbs 47g - Protein 10g

A delicious and super-simple dish that lends itself to a million interpretations and variations based on the best seasonal veggies. In the summer, you will choose tomatoes or cherry tomatoes, bell peppers, eggplants and zucchini, while in the winter you may prefer broccoli, cauliflower, kale. Let yourself be inspired by the greengrocer's stand!

In a deep skillet or wok, sautée the celery, onion and carrot, then add the veggies of your choosing. Season with chili pepper and salt and add a few chopped anchovy fillets for extra taste. While the veggies cook, add a few tablespoons of water if necessary.

In the meanwhile, cook the whole-grain pasta in boiling salted water.

When the pasta is ready, toss it in the pan with the veggies for a few minutes, and it's ready to go!

EGG AND SPINACH CASSEROLE

Ingredients for 4 servings:
10 oz fresh spinach (or 1 package frozen chopped spinach)
4 eggs
EVO oil
Salt and pepper

Prep time: 5 minutes - Cook time: 15 minutes total

Nutritional values per serving: Calories 266 - Fat 25g - Carbs 4g - Protein 11g

This dish only takes a few minutes to prepare and is a tasty idea to incorporate eggs in your healthy Mediterranean diet.

Preheat the oven to 180°C/375F.

Boil the spinach in a large pot of salt water, then drain them and arrange them in a casserole. Break the eggs over the spinach and season the whole thing with a drizzle of olive oil and a dash of salt and pepper.

Bake for five minutes or however long it takes for the eggs to appear thoroughly cooked.

Serve with a few slices of sourdough or whole-wheat bread.

TILAPIA TACOS WITH GREEK YOGURT

Ingredients for 4 servings:
4 corn taco shells or tortillas
1 lb tilapia fillets
1 cup Greek yogurt
2 green onions, chopped
½ cup fresh cilantro, chopped
1 lime, squeezed and zested
1 clove garlic, minced
1 head lettuce
2 large tomatoes, diced
3 tbsps EVO oil
Pepper, ground cumin and paprika

Prep time: 15 minutes - Cook time: 10 minutes

Nutritional values per serving: Calories 451 - Fat 22g - Carbs 27g - Protein 58g

A tasty dish where the lime and the spices combine perfectly with the Greek yogurt-based sauce and the fish's delicate taste. It works perfectly with any white fish fillets (tilapia, haddock, cod).
First of all, preheat the oven at 200°C/420F.
Prepare the fish by placing the fillets on a baking sheet. Combine the ground spices in a bowl and sprinkle them over the fish, then turn the fillets over and sprinkle the other sides as well. Put the fish in the oven and bake for 10 minutes or until the fish is well done through.

While the fish is cooking, take a large mixing bowl and mix the Greek yogurt with the chopped onions, cilantro, the minced garlic, the juice and zest from the lime.

Once the fish fillets are ready, break them apart with a fork. Assemble the tacos or tortillas by spreading the Greek yogurt sauce on them, adding the fish and topping with lettuce strips and diced tomatoes.

CHILI - GARLIC SPAGHETTI

Ingredients for 4 servings:
12 oz whole-wheat spaghetti
4 cloves of garlic, sliced
1 oz breadcrumbs
2 fresh chili peppers, crushed
4 tbsps EVO oil

Prep time: 5 minutes - Cook time: 15 minutes

Nutritional values per serving: Calories 277 - Fat 32g - Carbs 15g - Protein 8g

A traditional Italian lunch that just bursts with flavor and is just hot enough.
Heat up the olive oil in a skillet and add 3 cloves of garlic, sliced thin, and 2 crushed chili peppers. When the garlic is browned, add the breadcrumbs and toss for 2-3 minutes, being careful not to burn the breadcrumbs.
In the meanwhile, bring a large pot of salted water to a boil and cook the spaghetti in it; once they are cooked al dente, drain them and toss them in the skillet for a few minutes.
You can drizzle a bit more olive oil over the plates just before serving.

SHRIMP AND AVOCADO SALAD

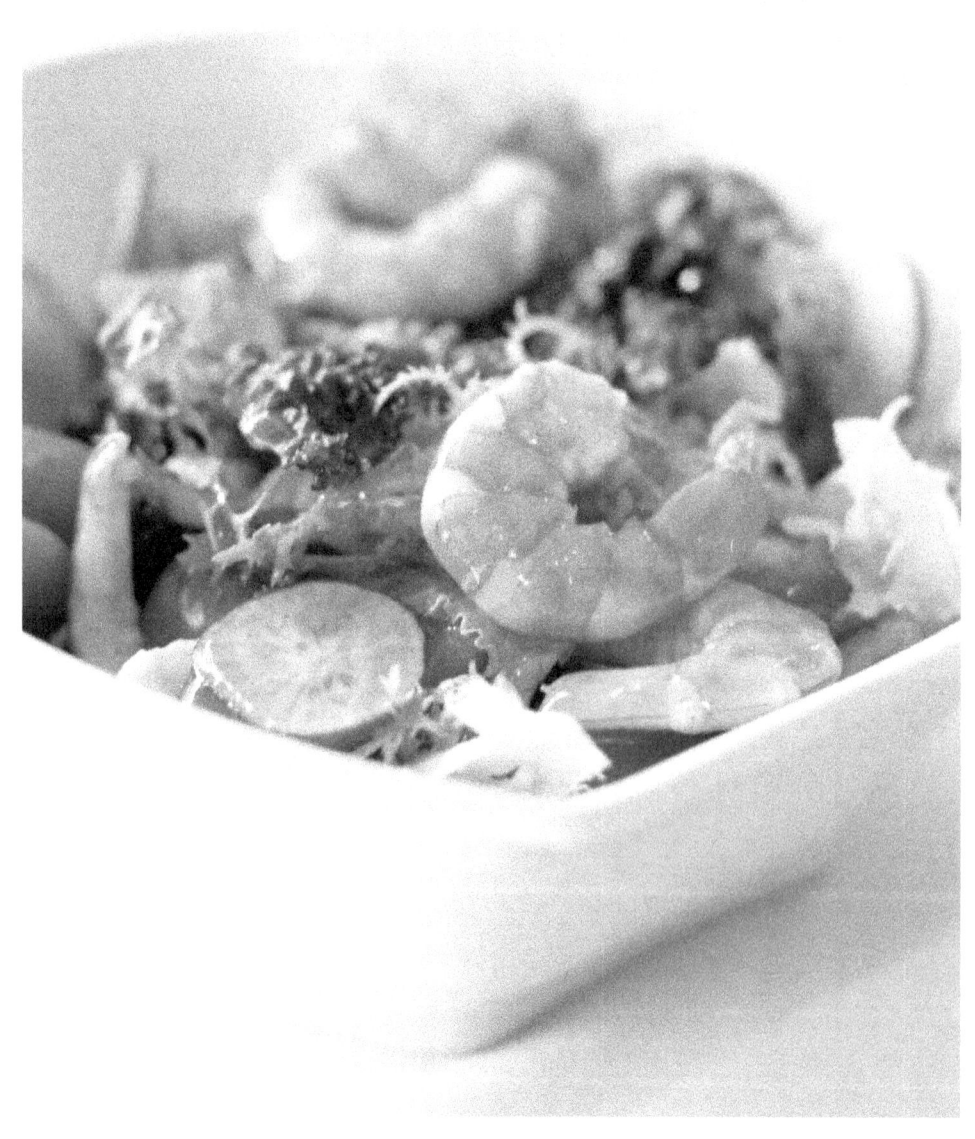

Ingredients for 4 servings:
16 small shrimp, cooked and chopped
2 avocados, diced
2 tomatoes, diced
2 scallions, chopped
1 cup crumbled feta cheese
1 lime, squeezed
EVO oil

Prep time: 5 minutes - Cook time: 15 minutes

Nutritional values per serving: Calories 422 - Fat 28g - Carbs 15g - Protein 30g

Full of nutrients and bursting with color and flavor, this wrap is an amazing idea for a simple springtime lunch! Also - did you know that shrimp are incredibly easy to cook? Read on to find out how!

To prepare the shrimp, cover the bottom of a large frying pan with a few tablespoons of EVO oil and place the pan over medium heat. As it heats up, tilt the pan to make sure the oil coats the whole surface. When the pan is warm, add the shrimp; if the pan is warm enough they will sizzle when touching its surface, otherwise you need a bit more heat, so try with one before adding them all!

Sauté the shrimp for approx. 10 minutes or until they are well cooked. It's easy to tell when they are ready: they will be completely opaque, pink in color, with bright-red tails. If some parts still appear grayish or translucent, cook for a while longer!

When the shrimp are ready, chop them up. Dice the avocados, the tomatoes, and the scallions; crumble the feta cheese in a bowl and squeeze the juice from one lime onto the feta.

Now you have all your ingredients ready, all you need to do is assemble the salad! Toss the ingredients in a bowl. Add seasoning to your taste (a dash of salt and freshly ground black pepper usually do the trick).

VEGGIE WRAP

Ingredients for 4 servings:
1 clove garlic
1 can chickpeas, rinsed and drained
1 lemon, squeezed
2 tbsps EVO oil
1 bunch fresh cilantro leaves, chopped
4 cups mixed greens
1 cucumber, sliced
2 cups cherry tomatoes, diced
1 red onion, sliced
4 wholemeal tortillas, wraps or pitas

Total time: 25 minutes

Nutritional values per serving: Calories 520 - Fat 13g - Carbs 70g - Protein 20g

A fulfilling vegetarian wrap that requires no cooking or baking!

First off, rinse and drain one can of chickpeas and place them in the food processor along with one clove of garlic, peeled and minced, 2 spoons of EVO oil, the juice from one lemon, salt and white pepper. Process until the mixture is smooth; remove it from the processor and place it in a mixing bowl, then add the chopped cilantro leaves and mix well.

In a separate bowl, combine mixed greens, one sliced or chopped cucumber, the cherry tomatoes and red onion. Dress with some EVO oil and black pepper or with a salad dressing of your choosing; toss the salad to combine well.

When you are ready to assemble the wraps, just spread a few tablespoons of the chickpea hummus-like sauce on each wrap, add the greens salad, roll up and serve.

The chickpea sauce can be prepped in advance and stored in the fridge for several days.

LEMON BARLEY SALAD

Ingredients for 4 servings:
2 cups uncooked barley
1 large lemon
1 cup of fresh basil leaves, chopped
2 ripe tomatoes, diced
2 carrots, shredded
¼ cup EVO oil
Salt and pepper to taste

Prep time: 15 minutes - Cook time: 15 minutes

Nutritional values per serving: Calories 463 - Fat 15g - Carbs 65g - Protein 14g

Just a few ingredients and a short prep time for a very tasteful and super healthy salad. This is perfect for an on-the-go lunch as well as for picnics, potlucks...
Zest the lemon and mix the zest with the lemon juice in a bowl. Add the EVO oil, salt, and pepper and mix it up, incorporating some air.
Cook the barley in salty water. When it's done al dente, drain it (but set aside 1 ladle of cooking water) and add it to the bowl with the sauce. Stir in the cooking water and let the barley soak up the sauce by placing it in the fridge to cool for 15 minutes. When it's cool, add the chopped basil leaves, tomatoes, and carrots. You may also add other ingredients of your choosing, such as other fresh herbs, mozzarella, or even grilled chicken! Extra tip: the longer you let it cool in the fridge before serving, the better it will taste.

OREGANO AND PARSLEY ZUCCHINI

Ingredients for 4 servings:
6-8 zucchini, sliced
2 cloves of garlic
EVO oil
Dried oregano
Fresh parsley leaves, chopped
Salt

Prep time: 5 minutes - Cook time: 40 minutes

Nutritional values per serving: Calories 170 - Fat 14g - Carbs 10g - Protein 4g

A simple and quick dish that is perfect to be used as a side for a main course of white meat or fish, or tossed with pasta, or even by itself over toasted bread.
Brown the garlic in hot EVO oil and slice the zucchini into thin rounds. Remove the garlic from the skillet and add the zucchini. Toss them for a few minutes on high heat. Then add the fresh parsley, lower the heat and let it cook for approx. 30 minutes, stirring occasionally. Season with salt and oregano and serve.

MASON JAR CHICKPEA SALAD

Ingredients for 4 servings:
Salad dressing of your choice
¼ cup EVO oil
2 cloves garlic, minced
1 small red onion
1 can chickpeas, drained and rinsed
2 cucumbers, chopped
1 head of lettuce, chopped
Fresh mint leaves, chopped
1 tsp dried oregano
Salt and black pepper to taste

Prep time: 15 minutes

Nutritional values per serving: Calories 344 - Fat 16g - Carbs 42g - Protein 11g

Mason jar salads are very in right now, and for a good reason: you can prep 4 servings (4 jars) at a time and have a ready-to-go meal at hand, that you can store in the fridge for up to 5 days in an airtight jar! This is just one of many types that you can prepare. The important thing is to layer the ingredients properly, with the dressing at the bottom and the salad leaves at the top.
First of all, pour your favorite salad dressing (such as vinaigrette, yogurt-based dressing...) into the bottom of the jar. Marinate the chopped onion in EVO oil for a few minutes, then add that to the jar too. On top of the dressing, layer the cucumbers, chickpeas, mint leaves and at last the lettuce. Sprinkle the

oregano, salt and freshly ground black pepper on top. All you'll have to do is pour the jar's contents into a large bowl and your salad will be perfectly seasoned and ready to eat!

BROCCOLI QUINOA SALAD

Ingredients for 4 servings:
1 ½ lbs broccoli
2 cloves garlic, minced
2 cups quinoa
1 onion, chopped
EVO oil
Salt and black pepper to taste

Prep time: 15 minutes - Cook time: 30 minutes

Nutritional values per serving: Calories 384 - Fat 5g - Carbs 68g - Protein 19g

Quinoa again, this time reinvented in a simple yet delicious lunch salad that will keep you going all afternoon. Being a basic recipe, it can be modified by adding a variety of different ingredients: crumbled feta cheese, chopped almonds or pistachios, fresh-squeezed lemon juice, spices...
Preheat the oven to 200°C/400F. Separate the broccoli florets and lay them in a single layer on a baking sheet. Peel and mince two cloves of garlic and sprinkle it over the broccoli florets. Drizzle with EVO oil and season with a dash of salt and black pepper. Place in the oven and bake for approx. 15 to 20 minutes.
While the broccoli roast, cook the quinoa. Combine 2 cups of quinoa with 4 cups of water in a wide saucepan and add salt; bring the water to a boil, then lower the heat, cover with a lid and let cook for 20 minutes or until the quinoa has absorbed most of the water.

When the broccoli florets are ready, chop them up and combine them with the quinoa in a large mixing bowl; add one onion, chopped thin, and a drizzle of EVO oil. If you wish to add other ingredients, now is the time to do it - but this recipe is already so tasty as it is!

Extra tip: both the quinoa and the roasted broccoli can be prepped in advance and stored in the fridge for days.

SEA BREAM WITH TOMATOES AND OLIVES

Ingredients for 4 servings:
2 cups cherry tomatoes
10 black olives
4 shallots
2 sea breams
4 cloves of garlic
EVO oil
Coarse salt
2 sprigs rosemary
Black pepper and dried oregano

Prep time: 20 minutes - Cook time: 30 minutes

Nutritional values per serving: Calories 305 - Fat 7g - Carbs 20g - Protein 40g

The sea bream is a very common fish in the Mediterranean diet, thanks to its lean yet tasty meat, rich in proteins, vitamins and minerals. This typical recipe pairs it with fresh tomatoes and olives for the ultimate Mediterranean taste.
Preheat the oven to 200°C/400F. Wash the tomatoes and cut them in half, without splitting them all the way. Pit the olives; clean the shallots and cut them in half.
Wash and clean the sea breams and stuff each one with a sliced clove of garlic, a pinch of coarse salt, a drizzle of olive oil, a rosemary sprig and a dash of black pepper. Wrap each fish in aluminum foil and arrange the tomatoes, olives, shallots and the remaining garlic (not peeled) around them. Season

with a drizzle of EVO oil, a dash of salt and pepper, and a handful of oregano. Close the foil around the fish and bake for 30 minutes.

Chapter 7: Dinner

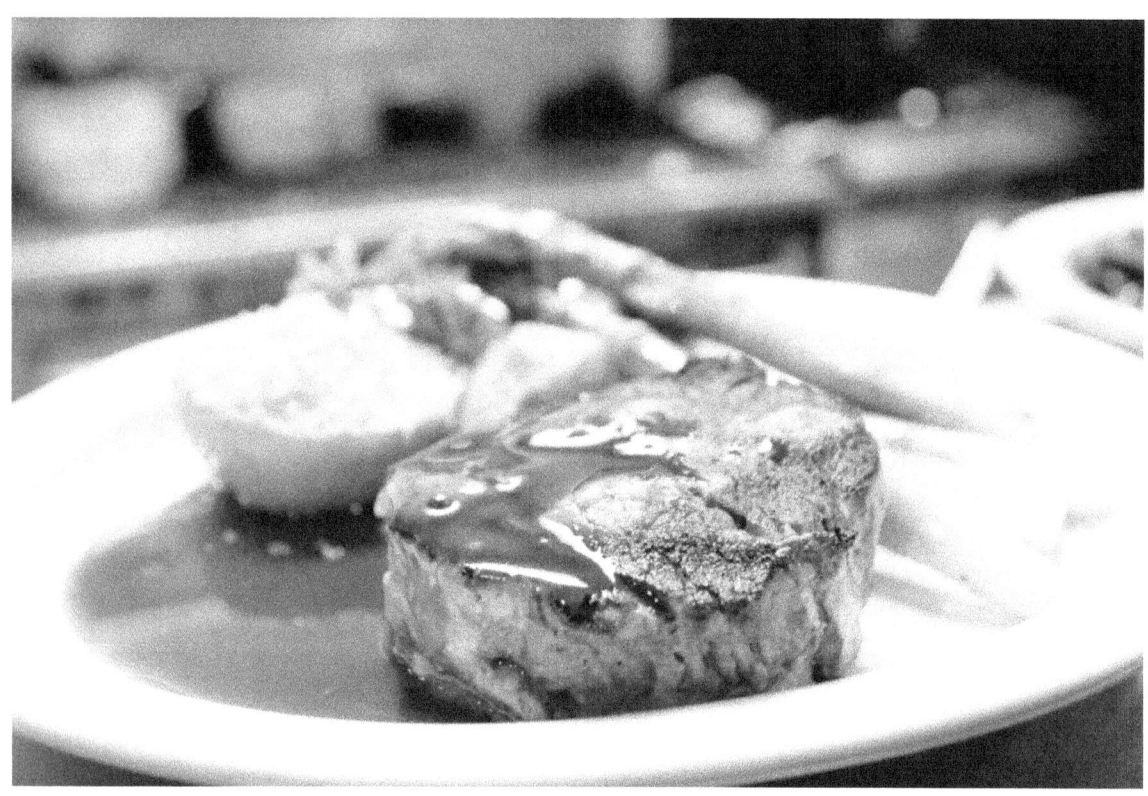

MOUSSAKA

Ingredients for 1 tin:
2 large eggplants (fresh, or sliced and frozen)
4 fresh ripe tomatoes, chopped
1 cup minced beef or red lentils
1 cup white sauce (béchamel)
2 cups various melting cheeses: mozzarella, feta

Prep time: 20 minutes - Cook time: 45 minutes

Nutritional values per serving: Calories 551 - Fat 32g - Carbs 31g - Protein 39g

A classic Greek and Balkan dish that can be prepared either with beef or with red lentils for a vegetarian version.

Preheat the oven to 180C/350F. Slice and fry the eggplants. Mix the minced beef (or red lentils) with the chopped tomatoes or the tomato sauce and add spices to taste. The resulting sauce must be thick, with no juice.

Make white sauce: melt 50g butter in a saucepan and mix 50g plain flour into it, stirring continuously to create a paste; in another saucepan, gently boil 500ml milk then gradually add it to the paste, and let cook for 5-10 minutes, stirring continuously. Melt the cheese in a saucepan (or microwave).
In a rectangular baking tin, create layers of eggplant, cheese, meat sauce and white sauce. Grate cheese on the top if you wish. Bake in preheated oven for approx 45 minutes.

CHICKPEA SOUP

Ingredients for 4 servings:
2 cans chickpeas, drained and rinsed
1 tbsp dried mushrooms
1 onion
Parsley
3 tomatoes, chopped
15 oz chard leaves
4 tbsps EVO oil
2 tbsps butter
Grated parmesan cheese

Prep time: 20 minutes - Cook time: 2 hours 15 minutes total

Nutritional values per serving: Calories 583 - Fat 25g - Carbs 70g - Protein 23g

A hearty soup that is just as delicious the next day. For extra substance, you can eat it with whole-wheat pasta (cooked separately).
Rinse and drain the chickpeas. Cook in salted water for about 2 hours (or 1 hour in a pressure cooker).
Brown the onions, parsley and mushrooms (previously soaked in tepid water for approx. 10 minutes) in a deep saucepan with the oil and butter until soft.
Add the tomatoes, chopped, and the chard leaves, previously chopped and blanched. Cook for a few minutes then add the chickpeas and cook for a further 10 minutes. Add water if necessary.
Serve topped with grated parmesan cheese.

BABAGANOUSH

Ingredients for 4 servings:
2 large eggplants
4 cloves of garlic
2 tbsps EVO oil
4 tbsps tahini (sesame sauce)
Juice from 2 lemons
2 tbsps finely minced parsley
Salt

Prep time: 20 minutes - Cook time: 30/45 minutes

Nutritional values per serving: Calories 223 - Fat 15g - Carbs 20g - Protein 6g

A typical Middle Eastern sauce or dish that exists in a million different versions, all of them equally tasty. Here is one of the "basic" interpretations.
Preheat the oven to its highest heat and bake the sliced eggplants for approx. 45 minutes, flipping them often. You can also use a gas or charcoal grill and place the eggplants directly over it; in that case, it will take approx. 30 minutes.
Once they are cooked through and very tender, slice them in two lengthwise and remove the flesh, placing it all in a stone mortar with the oil and the tahini.
Grind the mixture until soft and smooth. Chop the garlic finely and add it to the cream, then squeeze in the lemon juice and mix the cream.
Add salt to taste and garnish with minced parsley.
Serve with warm croutons or grilled bread slices.

RATATOUILLE

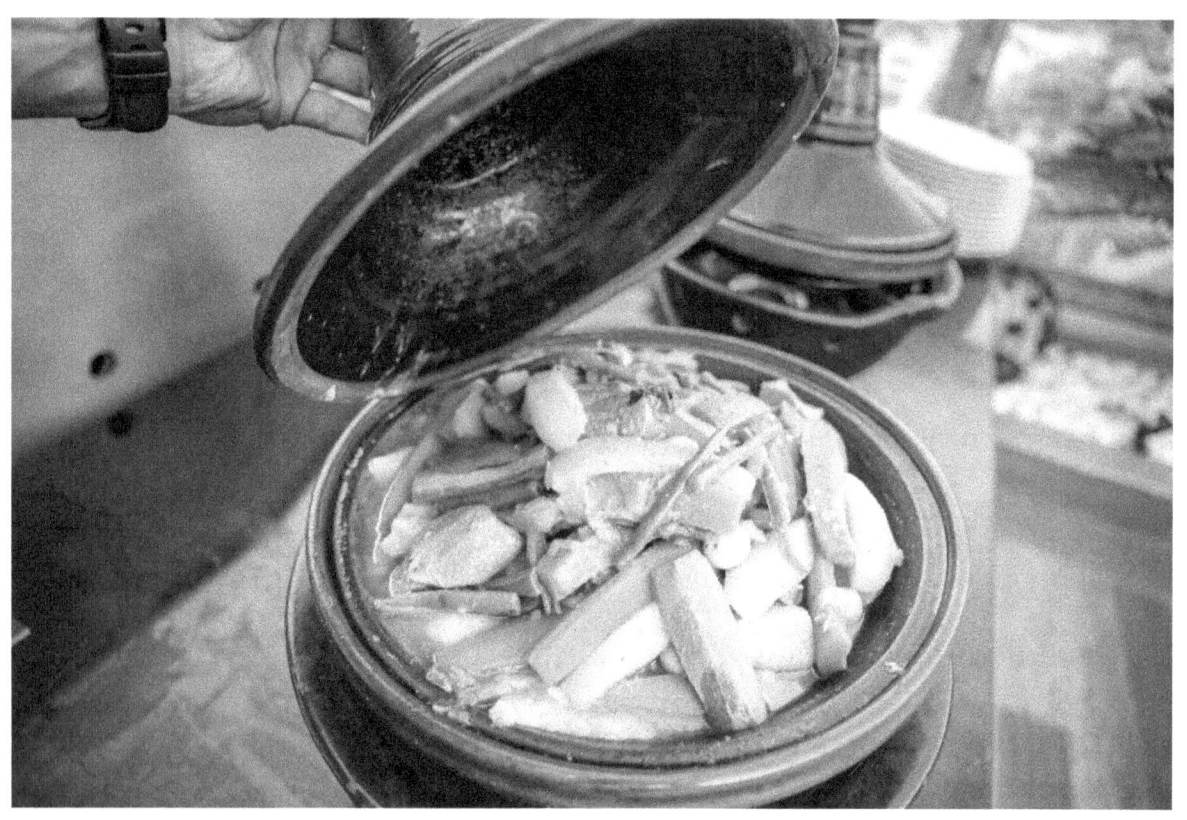

Ingredients for 4 servings:
4 large ripe tomatoes, diced
4 eggplants, diced
2 bell peppers, diced
4 zucchini, diced
2 onions, diced
6 cloves of garlic, minced
Basil leaves
6 tbsps olive oil
Salt, pepper

Prep time: 20 minutes - Cook time: 2 hours 30 minutes

Nutritional values per serving: Calories 418 - Fat 22g - Carbs 54g - Protein 11g

All the veggies in this colorful dish that bursts with flavor. It takes a while to cook, but it's worth it! Extra tip: make a larger dose and store in the fridge for the next few days. A leftover ratatouille lunch will brighten your day!

Pour half the oil in a lidded clay pot. Slice the onions thin and sweat them over low heat. Peel and slice the zucchini and eggplants, dice them and pan-fry them in a separate pot with the rest of the oil.
After a few minutes, transfer them to the pot with the onions, along with their cooking oil, and add the bell peppers, cleaned and diced. Pan-fry everything for 5 minutes then add in the chopped tomatoes, the minced garlic and the chopped basil leaves.

Season to taste, cover the pot and cook for approx. 2 hours, stirring every now and then to make sure it doesn't stick to the pan. Ratatouille tastes even better the day after you cook it!

KEFTETHES

Ingredients for 4 servings:
14 oz minced beef
7 oz breadcrumbs
1 egg
1 cup water
1 tbsp red wine vinegar
Fresh mint leaves, chopped
Oregano
Salt, pepper
Flour
Olive oil

Prep time: 15 minutes - Total time: 2 hours 30 minutes

Nutritional values per serving: Calories 400 - Fat 10g - Carbs 36g - Protein 38g

Typical Greek meatballs that can be made vegetarian by replacing the beef with cauliflower or even shredded carrots and bell peppers.

Lightly beat the egg and mix in the minced beef and the breadcrumbs, adding enough water to obtain a soft but thick mixture. Peel and chop the onions and sweat them in butter. Add the onions to the beef along with vinegar, oregano and mint leaves, and mix thoroughly. Leave to rest for 2 hours in a cool place. After 2 hours, form flattened balls with your hands and toss them in flour. Fry in olive oil until they brown then pat dry.

SPELT AND BEAN SOUP

Ingredients for 4 servings:
1 piece of celery, minced
1 carrot, minced or shredded
2 white onions, chopped
1 cup spelt
1 can beans (cannellini or borlotti)
6 sage leaves, whole
1 tbsp tomato paste
5 tbsps EVO oil
Salt and black pepper

Prep time: 10 minutes - Cook time: 1 hour 30

Nutritional values per serving: Calories 323 - Fat 19g - Carbs 34g - Protein 6g

A healthy, hearty and filling soup perfect for a winter night.

Place the beans in a large pot with one cup of water, one chopped onion and the sage leaves. When they are cooked, remove from the pot, divide them into two parts and mince one of the parts, then return it all to the pot. In another pot, sweat the other onion, the celery and the carrot in EVO oil and add the tomato paste. Cook for 15 minutes, then add the beans and their liquid.
After 10 more minutes add the spelt, season with salt and pepper and let cook for about 1 hour - the longer the better!

SUN-DRIED TOMATO AND GOAT CHEESE PASTA SALAD

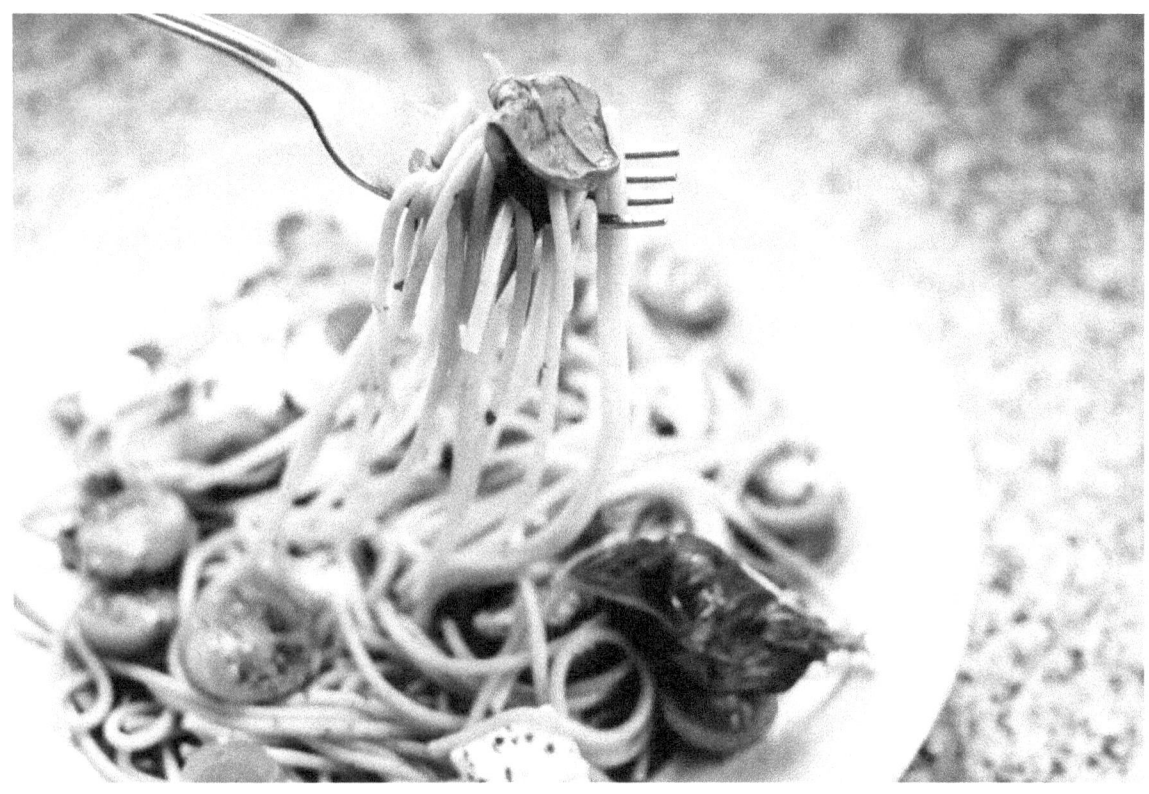

Ingredients:
½ cup EVO oil
1 cup fresh basil leaves
Juice from 1 lemon
1 clove garlic
Dried chili pepper
Salt to taste
14 oz short whole-wheat pasta
4-6 oz soft goat cheese

1 jar sun-dried tomatoes, chopped

Prep time: 15 minutes / Cook time: 10 minutes

Nutritional values per serving: Calories 657 - Fat 16g - Carbs 103g - Protein 27g

A bright and tasty pasta salad for a springtime dinner or picnic.

Boil a large pot of salted water and cook the pasta *al dente*. While it cooks, in a bowl, combine the olive oil, chopped basil leaves, lemon juice, garlic, salt and chili pepper and blend to make a sauce. Drain the pasta into a salad bowl and add the goat cheese and the basil-lemon sauce; add the sun-dried tomatoes and toss to combine. Any leftovers will make for a great packed lunch the next day!

CHICKEN GYROS

Ingredients for 4 servings:
8/12 chicken thighs, boneless and skinless
4 pcs pita bread or flatbread (store-bought or homemade)
4 tbsps olive oil
2 tbsps dried oregano
2 tbsps dried mint
1 tsp sweet paprika
1 tsp coriander
1 lemon, zest and juice
4 garlic cloves, crushed

For the tzatziki:
2 cups greek yogurt
1 cucumber
Fresh mint leaves, chopped
1 garlic clove, crushed
1 lemon, juice

For serving:
1 head of lettuce
2 large ripe tomatoes
1 red onion

Prep time: 30 minutes - Cook time: 25 minutes (plus resting time)

Nutritional values per serving: Calories 812 - Fat 33g - Carbs 28g - Protein 96g

Tender, flavor-soaked chicken served with salad and delicious tzatziki sauce.

First of all, marinate the chicken with all the marinade ingredients in a large bowl; mix well to make sure that all the thighs are covered in marinade. Leave to rest in the fridge for at least 4 hours, but the longer the better (you can marinate the chicken up to 48 hours in advance for maximum taste!).

Make the tzatziki by chopping up the cucumber (be sure to remove the seeds and squeeze any excess liquid) and combining it with the Greek yoghurt and the rest of the ingredients.

Arrange the chicken thighs onto skewers. Heat up the grill and place the skewers on a large roasting tin, so that there is some space underneath them. Cook the chicken in the grill for approx. 20 minutes, turning the skewers over halfway through.

In the meanwhile, heat up the pita bread in a frying pan.

When the chicken is done, remove it from the skewers and place it in the warm pita breads, along with some lettuce, sliced tomatoes, chopped onions and the tzatziki.

MEDITERRANEAN GAZPACHO

Ingredients for 4 servings:
2 cups cherry tomatoes
2 large ripe tomatoes
½ cup oil-preserved bell peppers
1 stalk celery
1 handful basil leaves
1 cup ricotta
2 tbsps EVO oil
2 Tropea onions
2 tbsps red wine vinegar
2 tbsps salt

For the croutons:
4 slices bread
1 tbsp EVO oil
Salt and pepper
1 tsp dried oregano

Total time: 30/40 minutes

Nutritional values per serving: Calories 181 - Fat 11g - Carbs 14g - Protein 4g

A refreshing version of the Andalusian gazpacho, bursting with Mediterranean flavors.

First off, dice the bread and place it in a wide frying pan (or on a baking sheet in the oven), seasoning oil, salt, pepper and oregano. Toast it until golden.

Wash and mince the celery and the tomatoes. Drain the bell peppers and chop them up too. Place all the vegetables in a food processor and season with olive oil, salt and vinegar. Blend until smooth. Strain the mixture to remove the tomato seeds.

Pour the gazpacho into a serving dish and garnish with Tropea onion rings and fresh basil leaves. Serve with the toasted croutons and dollops of ricotta cheese. The soup can be stored in the fridge (without the cheese and croutons) for several days and is also great as a leftover lunch.

SWORDFISH TARTARE

Ingredients for 4 servings:
2 swordfish fillets
2 cups Pachino tomatoes
2 shallots
1 tbsp capers
1 tbsp basil leaves
1 tbsp parsley leaves
1 tbsp mint leaves
1 tbsp marjoram leaves
1 lemon
2 tbsps EVO oil
Salt and black pepper

Total time: 15 minutes

Nutritional values per serving: Calories 200 - Fat 6g - Carbs 7g - Protein 29g

A simple, healthy dish whose secret lies in the balance of all the fresh herbs with the lemon emulsion.

Start by mincing the shallots, the capers and all the herbs on a cutting board. In a tall container, blend the lemon zest and juice with the EVO oil and season with salt and pepper. Whisk the mixture with a fork or an electric mixer. Cut the tomatoes into four parts, removing the seeds, then dice them. Defrost the swordfish fillets, remove the skin and dice them. In a mixing bowl, combine the fish with the herbs, the tomatoes, the capers and then season with the lemon emulsion right before serving. For extra flavor, you may also add a drizzle of soy sauce or tabasco.

CHICKEN COUSCOUS BOWL

Ingredients for 4 servings:
1 ½ cup uncooked couscous
1 cup Greek yogurt
1 ½ tbsps white wine vinegar
1 clove garlic, minced
12oz chicken meat, skinless and boneless, shredded
1 cup broccoli florets, chopped
1 cup cherry tomatoes, halved
1 red onion, sliced
Salt and pepper

Prep time: 20 minutes - Cook time: 20 minutes

Nutritional values per serving: Calories 420 - Fat 14g - Carbs 55g - Protein 40g

Simple bowls that you can adapt to whatever veggies you have at hand. You could also use salmon fillets instead of the chicken or leave it out entirely for a vegetarian alternative.

Pour 2 cups of water into a pot on high heat and bring to a boil. Pour the couscous into the boiling water, cover and let simmer for approx. 15 minutes. When it's done, drain and rinse with cold water, then drain again to avoid the grains sticking together.

Shred the chicken meat and sauté it in hot oil in a separate skillet, until it is nice and pink.

In a large mixing bowl, whisk the Greek yogurt with the vinegar and the garlic.

Divide the couscous into 4 medium-sized bowls. Chop or slice the vegetables and arrange them over the couscous, along with the chicken, then top with a few tablespoons of the Greek yogurt sauce.

ZUCCHINI ROLLS

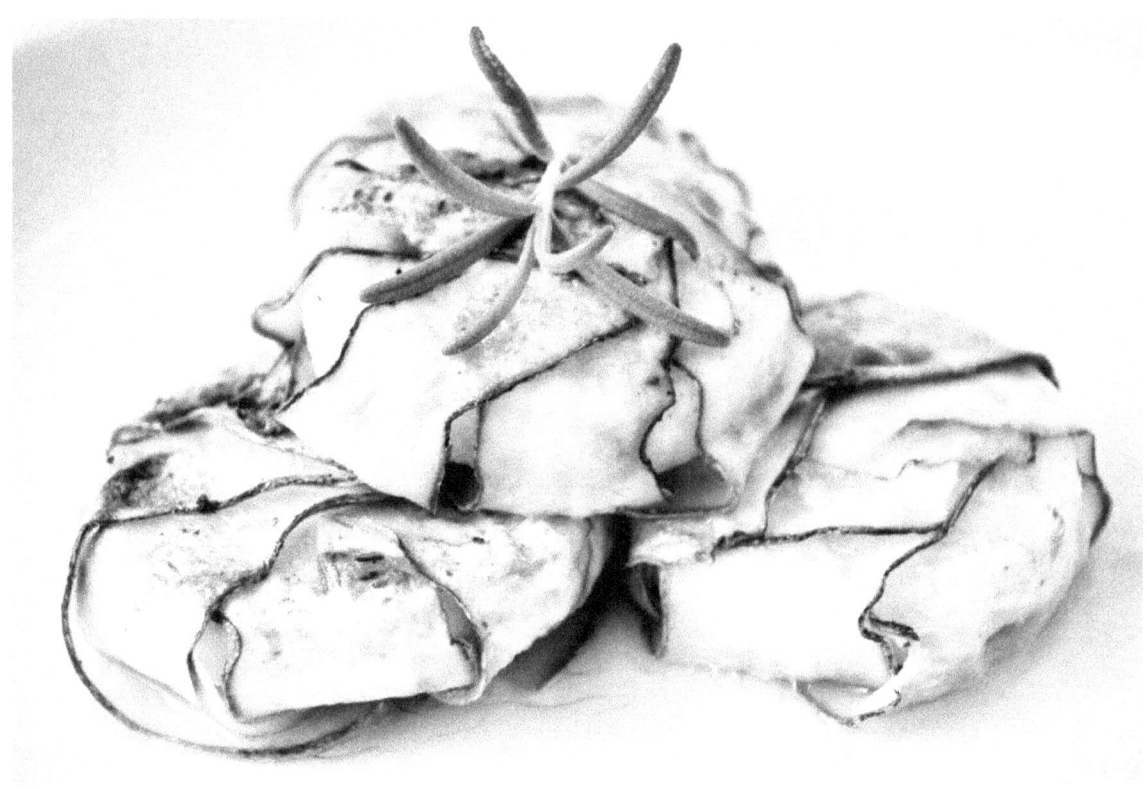

Ingredients for 4 servings:
2 large or 4 small zucchini
5 oz Parma ham
3 oz Edamer or Emmental cheese
1 egg
Breadcrumbs
Salt and EVO oil

Prep time: 10 minutes - Cook time: 20 minutes

Nutritional values per serving: Calories 181 - Fat 10g - Carbs 8g - Protein 16g

Even the pickiest veggie eaters won't be able to resist these tasty rolls!
Preheat the oven to 200°C/400F.
Slice the zucchini thin, lengthwise, and grill them. You may also do this in advance, eg. the day before. Slice the cheese and ham. Place a piece of cheese and some ham at the center of each zucchini slice and roll them up.
Beat the egg with some salt. Once all the rolls are ready, dip them in the egg then coat with breadcrumbs. Arrange the rolls in a baking tin and drizzle with EVO oil. Put in the oven and bake for approx. 20 minutes, until they appear nice and brown. Equally delicious the next day!

MEDITERRANEAN NACHOS

Ingredients for 4 servings:
1 large bag whole-wheat nachos
2 ripe tomatoes, chopped
1 red onion, chopped
1 cucumber, chopped
2 tbsps EVO oil
2 tbsps red wine vinegar
1 can chickpeas, rinsed and drained
2 tbsps tahini
1 lemon, squeezed
1 clove garlic
1 cup Greek yogurt
1 cup mozzarella cheese, shredded
Parsley and mint leaves, fresh or dried
Salt and pepper

Prep time: 15 minutes - Cook time: 10 minutes

Nutritional values per serving: Calories 415 - Fat 22g - Carbs 42g - Protein 17g

This Mediterranean take on a nacho plate makes for a lovely appetizer for a dinner with friends, or a great snack plate.
First, preheat the oven to 180°C/375F.
Grab your food processor and use it to blend the tomatoes, cucumber, onion, 1 tbsp oil and 1 tbsp vinegar. When your "salsa" is smooth, let it cool in the fridge for 30 minutes to 1 hour.

While it cools, make the hummus by blending the chickpeas (rinsed and drained) with the tahini, lemon juice and minced garlic. You don't want the hummus to be too thick because you will have to drizzle it over the nachos.

In a large mixing bowl, whisk the Greek yogurt with 2 tbsps lemon juice, the mint and parsley leaves, 1 tbsp EVO oil and 2 tbsps red wine vinegar.

Extra tip - all the sauces (the salsa, the hummus and the Greek yogurt mix) can be prepared in advance and stored in airtight containers in the fridge for a few days.

Then, arrange the nacho chips on a baking sheet; sprinkle the shredded mozzarella over them and stick in the oven for a few minutes, until the cheese begins to melt.

Top the nachos by drizzling the salsa, the yogurt mix and the hummus. Serve garnished with lemon slices and a drizzle of EVO oil.

KALE, MUSHROOM AND ONION FRITTATA

Ingredients for 4 servings:
2 large eggs
1 cup kale leaves, chopped
1 cup cremini mushrooms, sliced
1 white onion, sliced
2 cloves garlic
EVO oil
1 tsp paprika
Salt and pepper

Prep time: 10 minutes - Cook time: 15 minutes

Nutritional values per serving: Calories 290 - Fat 22g - Carbs 5g - Protein 18g

A yummy frittata, with all the benefits that wonderful kale can give.
Break the eggs in a large mixing bowl and beat them with salt, pepper and paprika, using a fork.
Cover the bottom of a frying pan with EVO oil and heat the oil; when it's ready, toss the onion and the mushrooms and sauté them for a few minutes, until the mushrooms start to brown. Then toss in the roughly chopped kale leaves and cook until they wilt.
Pour the egg mixture in the skillet and stir it in well, tilting the pan so it covers the whole bottom and incorporates all the veggies. After a few minutes or so, when the eggs are not runny anymore, you will have to flip the frittata to cook the bottom side as well; you can easily do this by placing a large plate over the skillet (the plate must be wider in diameter than the skillet itself) and turning

the pan over, then removing the plate and sliding the frittata back into the skillet.

Serve alone or with crumbled feta or goat cheese.

TOMATO AND MUSHROOM ROAST WITH BURGUL

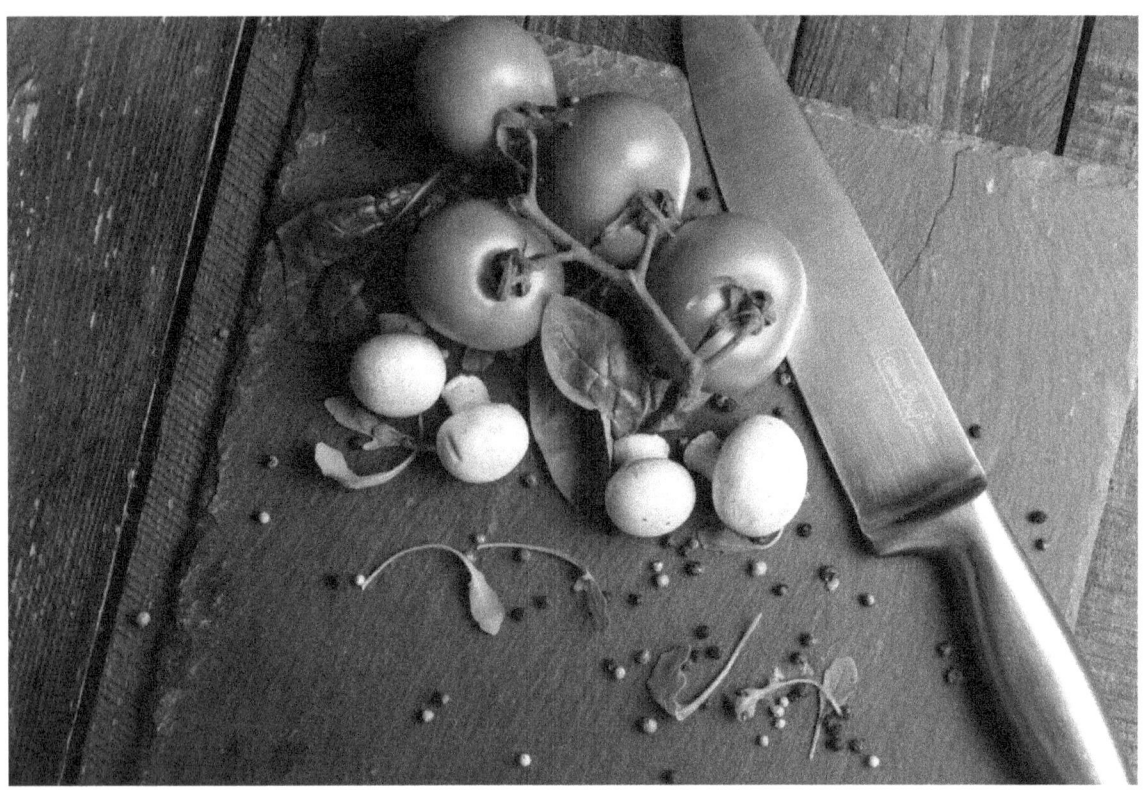

Ingredients for 4 servings:
4 cups cherry tomatoes, halved
2 cups champignon mushrooms, halved
½ cup fresh thyme leaves
4 cloves garlic, minced
Salt and pepper
2 tbsps balsamic vinegar
4 tbsps EVO oil
2 cups fine bulgur

Prep time: 10 minutes - Cook time: 35 minutes

Nutritional values per serving: Calories 422 - Fat 16g - Carbs 65g - Protein 12g

Preheat the oven to 180°C/375F.

Wash the cherry tomatoes and the mushrooms and cut them in half (quarters if they are large). Place them in a large mixing bowl with 1 tbsp olive oil, the thyme leaves, and a dash of salt and fresh-ground black pepper. Toss so as to coat the tomatoes and mushrooms with the thyme leaves.

Arrange the tomatoes, cut-side down, and the mushrooms, in a single layer, on a large baking sheet coated with parchment paper.

Place in the oven and let them roast for 30/35 minutes, until the veggies are soft and caramelized. When they are cooked, drizzle the balsamic vinegar over them.

Soak or cook the bulgur according to the instructions on the packaging and serve in a bowl, topped with the roasted veggies.

The vegetables can be prepped and roasted in advance and refrigerated in an airtight container for up to 5 days. Just reheat them in the oven when you are ready!

CAULIFLOWER PIZZA BASE

Ingredients for 1 pizza:
1 large head cauliflower
1 egg
1 cup Parmesan or mozzarella cheese, shredded
Mixed dried herbs of your choosing (oregano, basil, marjoram...)
Garlic powder, salt, pepper

Total time: 1 hour

Nutritional values per serving (base only): Calories 190 - Fat 8g - Carbs 12g - Protein 17g

A diet-proof alternative to a pizza crust that you can top with all the ingredients you like: tomato sauce, mozzarella, fresh tomatoes or bell peppers, ham, eggs, whatever!
Preheat the oven to 180°C/375F.
Clean the cauliflower and separate its florets. Place them in a food processor and process until the texture starts to resemble grains of rice. Transfer to a baking tin and bake in the oven for approx. 15 minutes. Remove from the oven, let cool for a while then strain any excess water by squeezing and mashing the cauliflower in a strainer or cloth. In a mixing bowl, combine the cauliflower with the egg, cheese and herbs.
Flatten out in a pizza tin and bake in the oven for 20 minutes, then carefully flip it over and bake for a few more minutes on the other side. You can then add your toppings of choice and place in the oven for a few more minutes to cook.

BAKED SPINACH TURKEY MEATBALLS

Ingredients for 4 servings:
2 cups spinach
4 cloves garlic
2 cups ground turkey meat
1 cup mozzarella cheese, shredded
½ cup breadcrumbs
1 cup whole-wheat orzo
2 red bell peppers, diced
2 carrots, diced
1 red onion, diced
2 tbsps EVO oil
Salt and pepper

Prep time: 20 minutes - Cook time: 25 minutes

Nutritional values per serving: Calories 550 - Fat 25g - Carbs 46g - Protein 38g

Whole-grain meets lean turkey and vegetables in this delicious meatball bowl. Basically all your Mediterranean diet nutrients in a single dish!
Preheat the oven to 200°C/400F.
Place the spinach in the food processor along with the garlic cloves and pulse for a few minutes. If you prefer to o it by hand, mince the spinach and garlic very thin.
In a large mixing bowl, combine the turkey met, the cheese, spinach and breadcrumbs and season to your liking. If the mixture is too dry, add a few more tablespoons EVO oil, or one egg. If it is too dry, add some more breadcrumbs. When the mixture has the right texture, roll it into balls using

your hands (you might want to coat your hands with breadcrumbs to avoid it sticking to your skin). Form 16-20 meatballs, depending on the size. Arrange them on a baking sheet and bake for 20 minutes.

While they bake, bring a large pot of salted water to a boil, then toss in the orzo and cook for 8 minutes or according to cooking instructions. Drain and put back into the same pot.

Dice and chop the bell peppers, the carrots and the onion and toss them in the pot with the orzo. Let cook for a few minutes then season with EVO oil, salt, pepper, and a drizzle of lemon juice.

Serve the meatballs with the orzo and garnish with fresh basil leaves.

ARTICHOKE AND TOMATO FISH BAKE

Ingredients for 4 servings:
4 cod fillets (any white fish will do)
1 yellow onion, chopped
4 cloves garlic
6 ripe tomatoes
14oz artichoke hearts
4oz green olives
2 tbsps capers
½ cup fresh basil leaves
3 tbsps EVO oil
Salt and pepper

Prep time: 15 minutes - Cook time: 30 minutes

Nutritional values per serving: Calories 300 - Fat 14g - Carbs 23 - Protein 26g

One more way to incorporate fish into your diet, where the white fish fillets are paired with tasty, juicy artichokes and olives.
Preheat the oven to 180°C/375F.
Cover the bottom of a large oven-safe skillet with olive oil. Tilt the pan so as to spread the oil evenly. Chop the onions. When the oil is warm, toss in the onions and the garlic, peeled but whole; sweat the onions and garlic until the garlic starts to brown. Toss the chopped tomatoes into the skillet. Season with salt and pepper and add the fresh basil leaves. Cook for 3-4 minutes then remove from heat.
Add the fish on top of the sauce.

If you are using canned artichoke hearts, drain them and then roughly chop them. If you are using fresh artichoke hearts, just slice them in half. You may also choose to leave them whole. Lay them in the skillet between and around the fish fillets. Add the olives and capers.

Drizzle the whole thing with EVO oil. Put the skillet in the oven and bake for approx. 20 minutes (more or less, depending on the size of the fillets).

When it is done, garnish with basil leaves and serve.

Thank you for choosing and reading this book. We hope it was useful and able to provide you with a thorough overview of the Mediterranean diet, its lifestyle, its dos and don'ts. We hope this book has helped you understand more about this diet and given you the tools to set off on further research, to learn about the background of this diet and the food pyramid it is based on. Please remember, however, not to undergo any significant lifestyle or dietary changes without consulting your GP as there may be contraindications to certain elements. If this isn't your case, the Mediterranean diet will surprise you with its beneficial effects on your health, including but not limited to improving the appearance of your skin, lowering your cholesterol levels, helping prevent the onset of type 2 diabetes... all this in addition to losing weight!

With the Mediterranean diet, it is not necessary to count every single calorie you are eating; you will not need to feel deprived or starved, or to ban certain foods you love from your diet. Sticking to the food pyramid we mentioned at the beginning of this book will help you establish healthier eating habits with little effort. Remember to choose smaller portions than you might be used to, to take your time to cook and eat, and to choose healthy snacks like nuts or fruit rather than sugary snacks or soda drinks. You are allowed to eat a great variety of food; just try to limit your intake of red meats, sugar, etc. in favor of fish, fresh fruit and vegetables.

Please consider that your eating habits alone are not enough to adjust your lifestyle dramatically; it is vital to include physical activity in your daily routine. For instance, without necessarily having to hit the gym every day of the week, you could try getting into the habit of walking or riding a bicycle instead of driving to work or to run your daily errands... Any small amount of physical activity is enough to spur your metabolism and help you burn calories.

The recipes we have provided in this book should be able to give you inspiration and get you into the habit of planning and prepping your meals, choosing high-quality, local and seasonal ingredients, and overall stocking up on the "right" types of food.

You will hopefully be able to switch to this healthier lifestyle and eating regime, without too much effort.

Please don't hesitate to leave a review if you have appreciated this book or found useful information in it!

Author email:

eathealtyeat@gmail.com

Visit the author's facebook page:

https://www.facebook.com/EatingHealtyEating

www.ingramcontent.com/pod-product-compliance
Lightning Source LLC
Chambersburg PA
CBHW080408290526
45791CB00008BA/2195